Crohn's Disease - Recent Advances

Edited by Monjur Ahmed

Published in London, United Kingdom

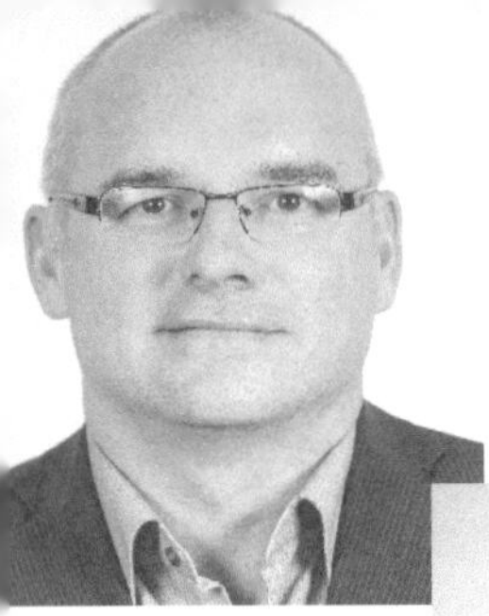
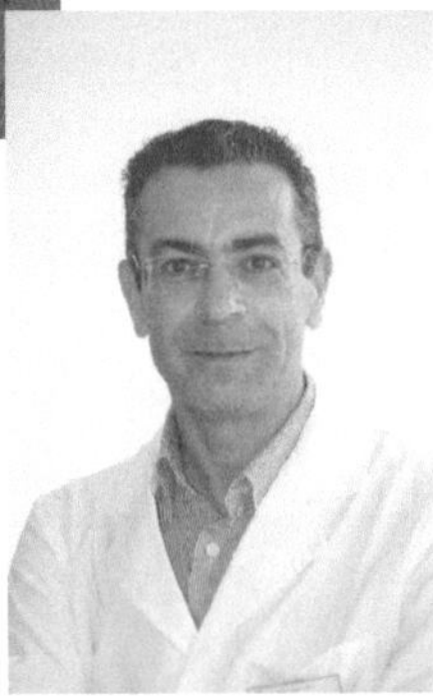
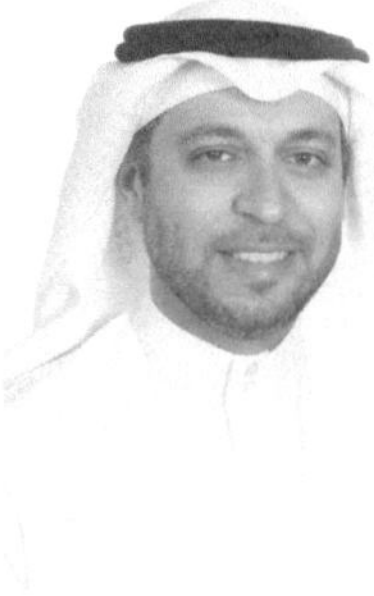
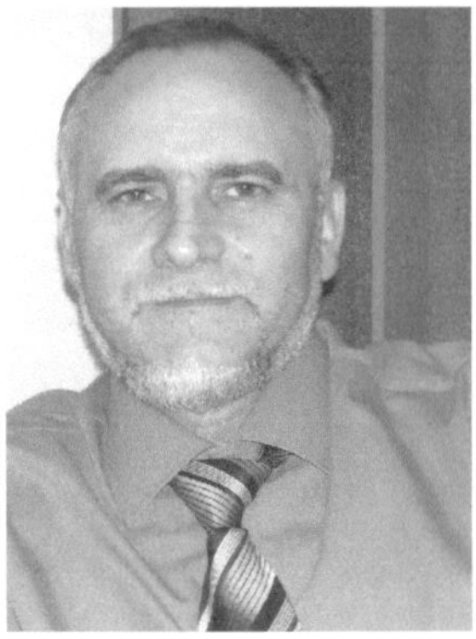
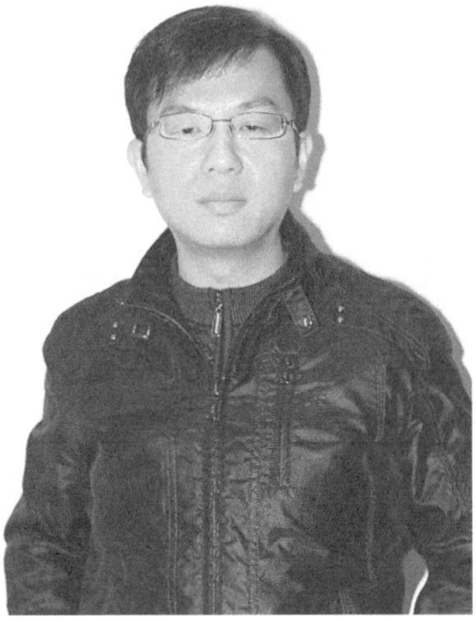
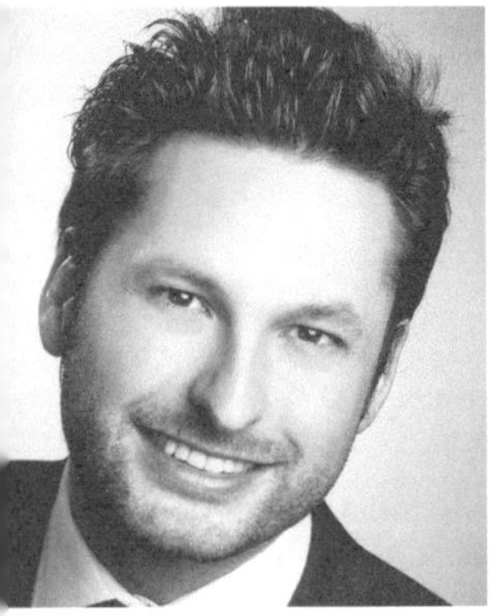
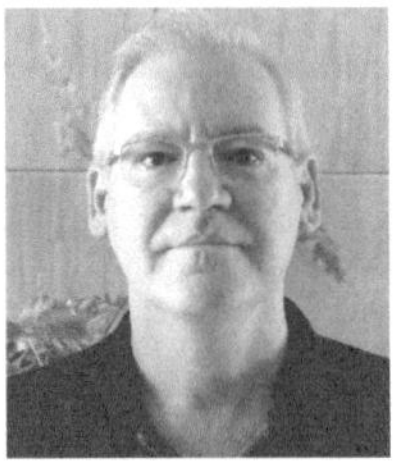

IntechOpen

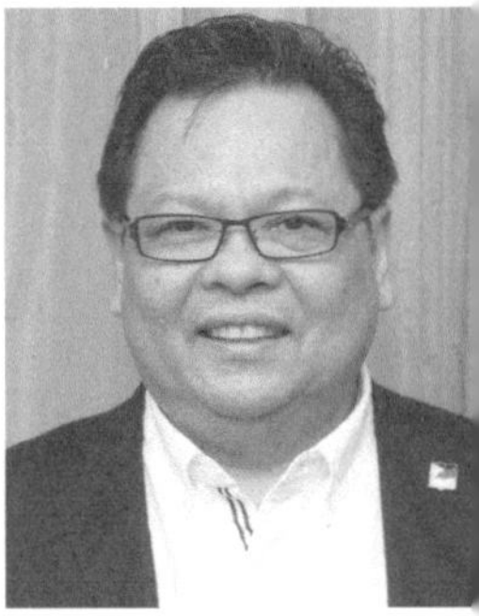
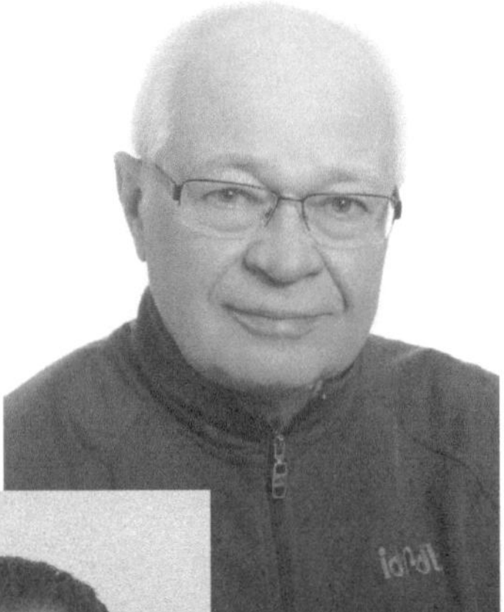
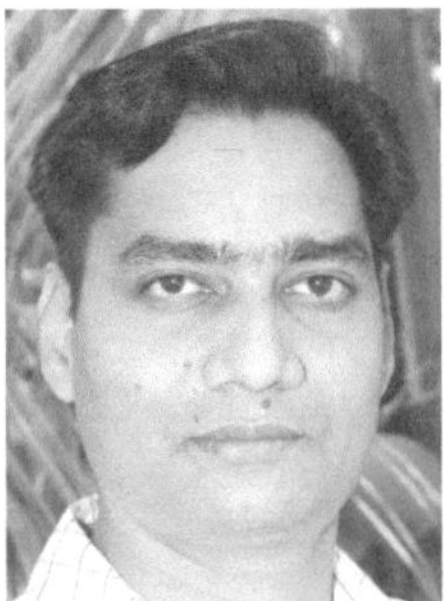
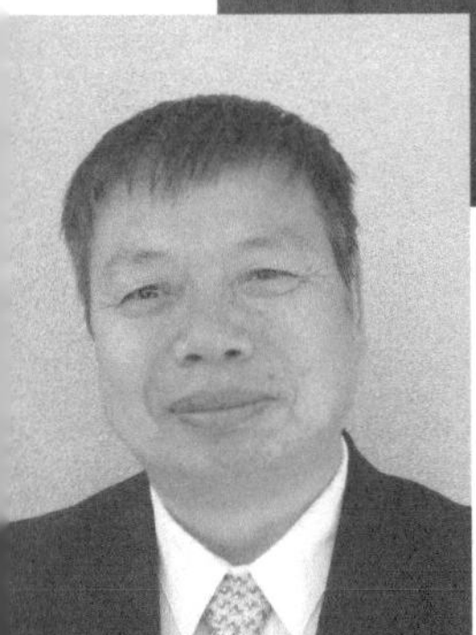
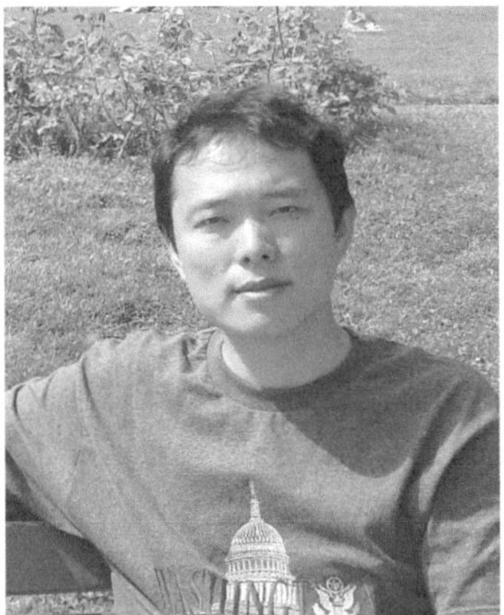
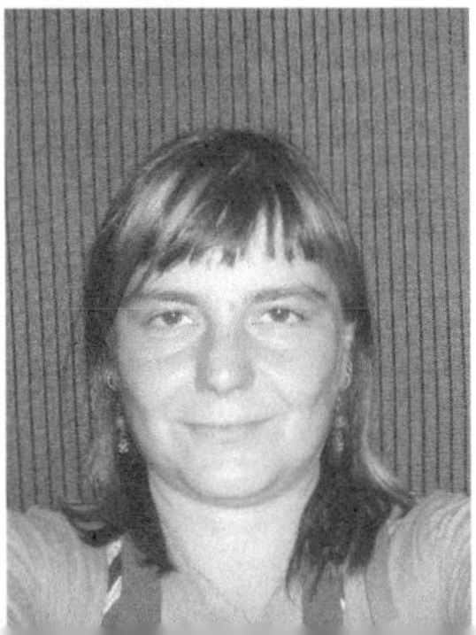

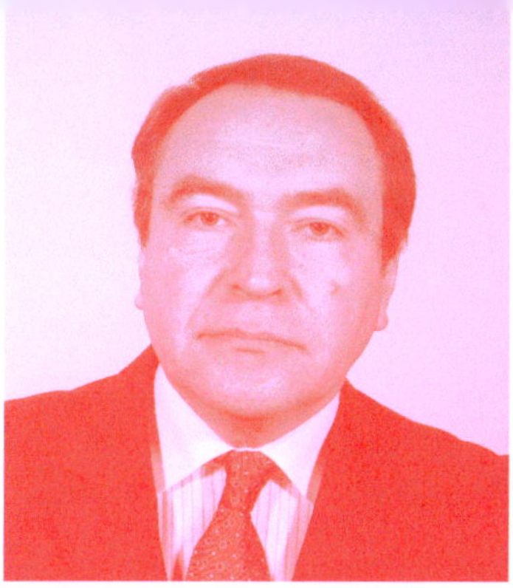
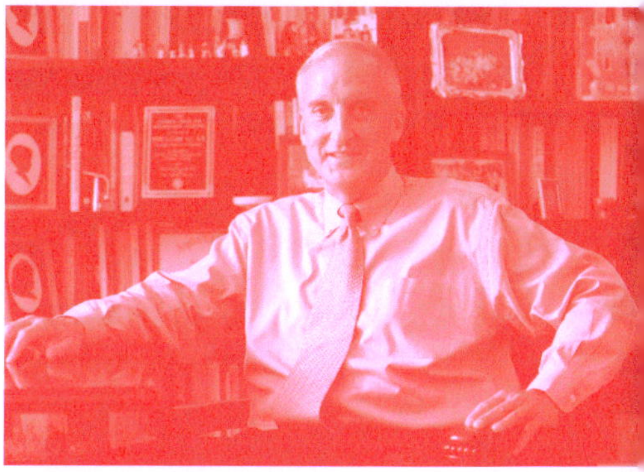
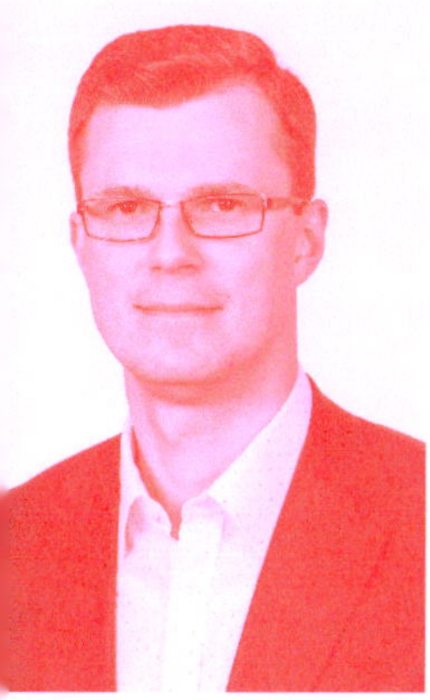
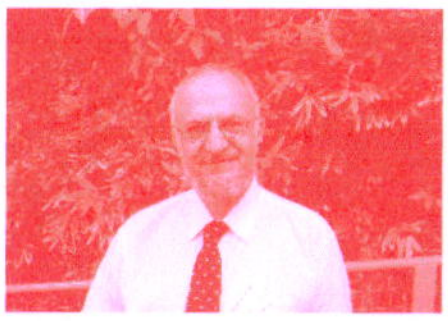
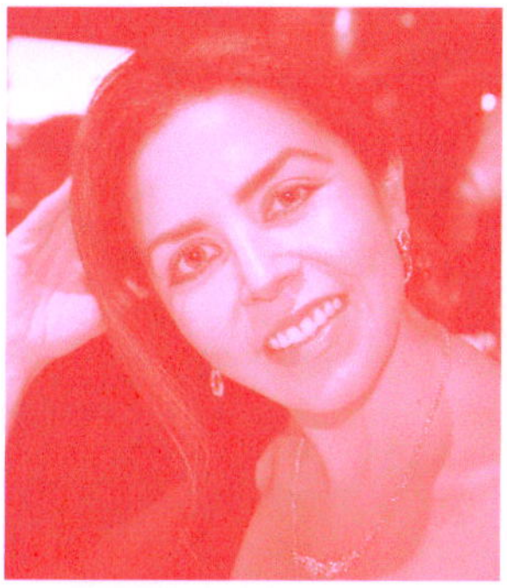

Supporting open minds since 2005

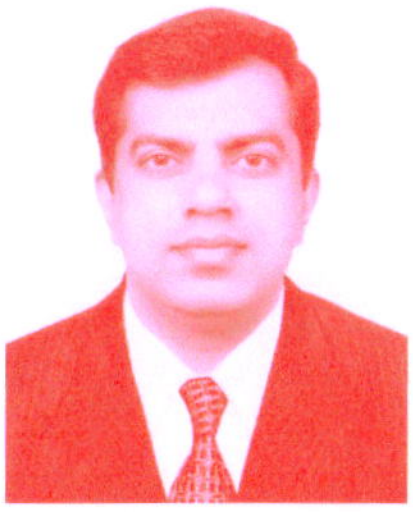
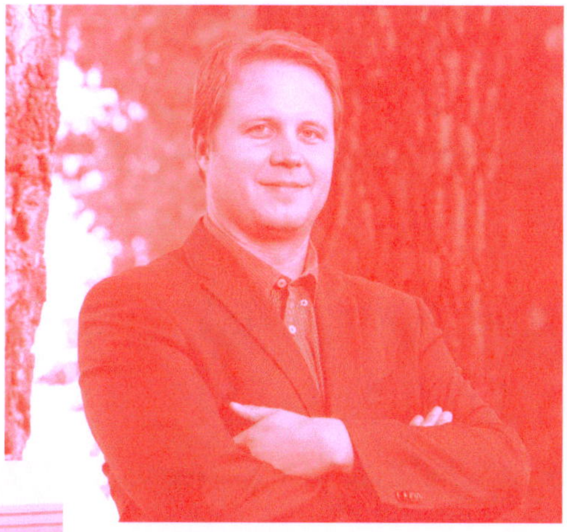
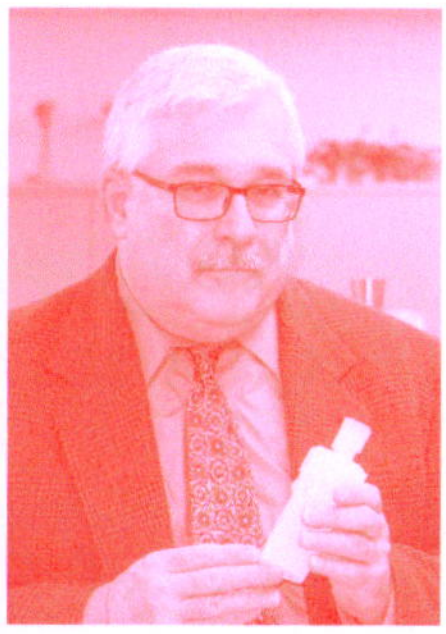
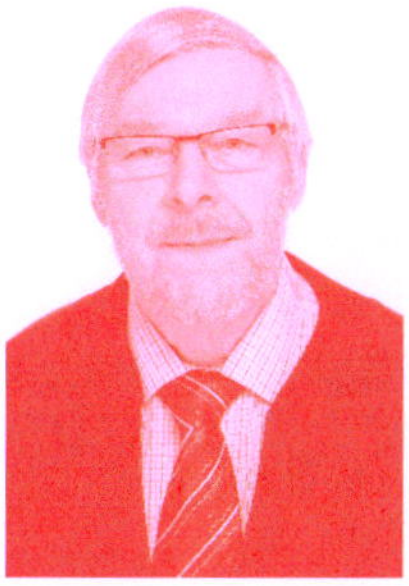
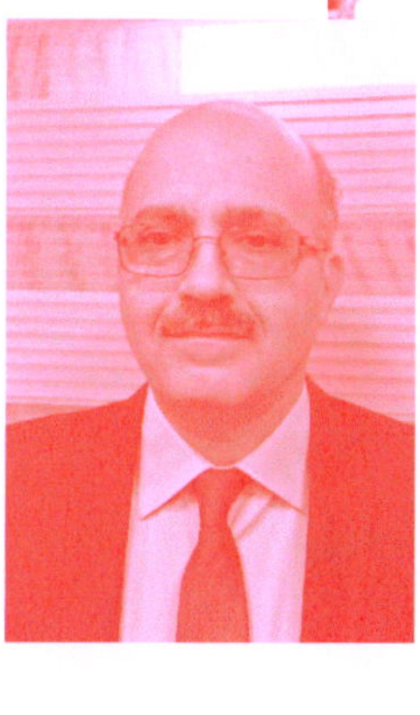
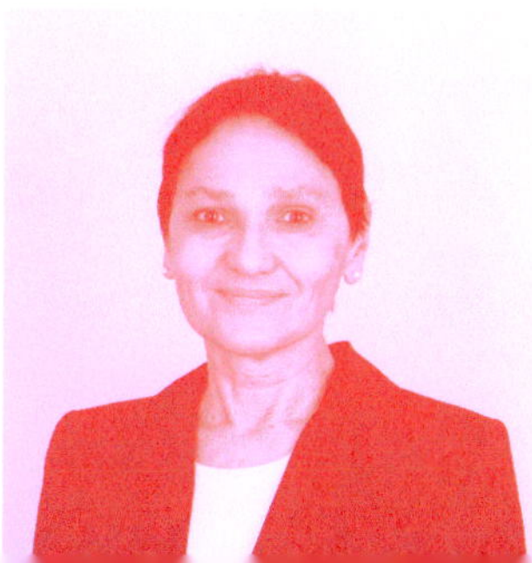
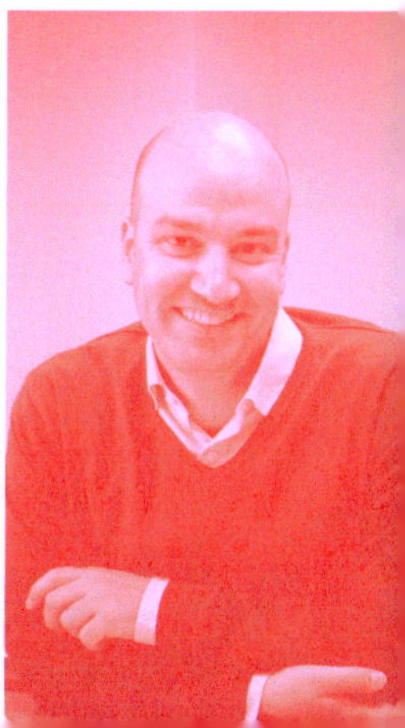

Crohn's Disease - Recent Advances
http://dx.doi.org/10.5772/intechopen.91501
Edited by Monjur Ahmed

Contributors
Daniel Vasile Balaban, Anjana Bali, Monika Rani, Xiaomei Wang, Siyi Lv, Mei Li, Huangan Wu, Luyi Wu, Evgen Benedik, Rok Orel, Darja Urlep, Anija Orel, Monjur Ahmed, Mariana Jinga

First published in London, United Kingdom, 2021 by IntechOpen
IntechOpen is the global imprint of INTECHOPEN LIMITED, registered in England and Wales, registration number: 11086078, 5 Princes Gate Court, London, SW7 2QJ, United Kingdom
Printed in Croatia

British Library Cataloguing-in-Publication Data
A catalogue record for this book is available from the British Library

Additional hard and PDF copies can be obtained from orders@intechopen.com

Crohn's Disease - Recent Advances
Edited by Monjur Ahmed
p. cm.
Print ISBN 978-1-83968-170-7
Online ISBN 978-1-83968-171-4
eBook (PDF) ISBN 978-1-83968-172-1

Meet the editor

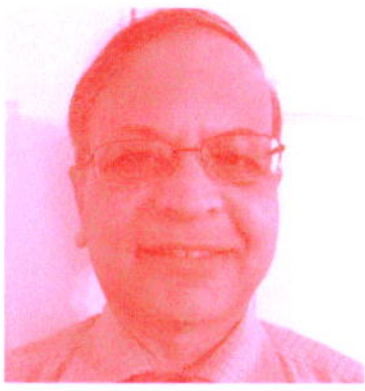

Monjur Ahmed, MD, FRCP, is an Associate Professor of Medicine at Thomas Jefferson University, Philadelphia, Pennsylvania, USA. He has been a practicing gastroenterologist for twenty-two years. He has a special interest in inflammatory bowel disease, eosinophilic esophagitis, gastrointestinal motility, and dysphagia. He also serves as an editor in chief of the *World Journal of Gastrointestinal Oncology*.

Contents

Preface

Crohn's disease is a chronic inflammatory disease of the gastrointestinal tract with many extra-intestinal features. Patients suffer from chronic symptoms with relapses and remissions. There are many recent advances in the treatment of this debilitating disease. This book discusses the extra-intestinal manifestations of Crohn's disease, recent advances in the diagnosis and management of Crohn's disease, and different treatment modalities including the role of leucocyte apheresis, parenteral nutrition, and Chinese medicine. This book is a good reference for gastroenterologists, internal medicine doctors, and primary care physicians who diagnose and manage Crohn's disease.

Monjur Ahmed
Associate Professor,
Thomas Jefferson University,
Philadelphia, Pennsylvania, USA

Dedication

I dedicate this book to my sister Masuma Jasmin Jhima.

Chapter 1

Introductory Chapter: Crohn's Disease - Recent Advances

Monjur Ahmed

1. Introduction

Crohn's disease and ulcerative colitis are the two main forms of inflammatory bowel disease (IBD). While ulcerative colitis mainly causes mucosal inflammation of the rectum and the colon, Crohn's disease is characterized by transmural inflammation of the gastrointestinal tract anywhere from the mouth to the anus and granuloma formation in about 30% of cases. Crohn's disease can also cause deep ulcers, penetrating ulcers, stricture, fistula, abscess, perforation, malabsorption and perianal disease. Although both forms of IBD can cause extra-intestinal manifestations and malignancy, Crohn's disease is, in fact, a much more severe disease and patients' sufferings can be relentless if the disease is not under control. The natural course of Crohn's disease is chronic inflammation with relapse and remission. As it affects mostly young population in the 20s and 30s, their prime time of life is hampered. So patients suffering from Crohn's disease always want to avoid any relapse and be in long-term remission. The exact etiology of Crohn's disease is unknown. Genetics, environmental factors (smoking, anxiety, depression, stress) and altered gut microbiota play important roles in disrupting the immune homeostasis that results in uncontrolled inflammation of the gut. A systematic review found that the prevalence of Crohn's disease was 319 cases per 100,000 people and the annual incidence was 20.2 cases per100,000 persons-year in the United States [1]. It is more commonly seen in the white population in the Western world, but any person of any ethnicity can be affected. It is slightly more common in females than in males. The incidence and prevalence of Crohn's disease have been increasing globally. Kochar et al. found that United States born Asians and Asian immigrants suffer from more perianal and ocular Crohn's disease compared with white Americans [2].

There are various laboratory, imaging and endoscopic studies available to diagnose and assess the severity of Crohn's disease. Crohn's Disease Activity Index (CDAI) and Harvey-Bradshaw Index (HBI) are commonly used to assess the activity of the disease. Classically, Crohn's disease is divided into mild, moderate and severe disease. There are various immunomodulatory [6-mercaptopurine (6-MP), azathiopurine (AZA), methotrexate (MTX), and janus kinase (JAK) inhibitors] and biologic agents (anti-tumor necrosis factor, anti-integrin, IL-12/IL-23 inhibitors and biosimilars) available at the present time for induction of remission and maintenance of remission of Crohn's disease. Mild Crohn's disease is generally treated by a short course of budesonide followed by maintenance with 6-MP, AZA or MTX. Moderate to severe disease is treated with systemic corticosteroid followed by biologic agents with or without immunomodulatory agents. Primary non-response and secondary loss of response to the biologic agents and immunomodulators are not uncommon. These unfavorable outcomes can be evaluated by therapeutic monitoring of trough levels of drugs, measuring anti-drug antibodies (for anti-TNF agents) and metabolite levels (for thiopurines) so that appropriate management strategy can be taken [3]. The goal of treatment is not only clinical and endoscopic remission but also mucosal healing. Although many patients are able to maintain long-term remission, the treatment options are not optimal considering their efficacy rate and side effect profile. As a result, many clinical trials are ongoing for better control of Crohn's disease. Many biologic agents are in the pipeline to be released into the market. Many patients ultimately need surgery when medical therapy fails and when complications occur. Fortunately, the surgery rate in Crohn's disease is decreasing. A population-based time-trend analysis showed that the incidence rates for surgery in Crohn's disease had been decreasing by about 8.4% each year from 1996 to 2013 [4]. Unfortunately, surgical intervention is not curative and patients still need to be on immunosuppressive or biologic agents to prevent recurrence of the disease. Preventive care is an important aspect of management of Crohn's disease. Because of immune dysregulation, patients are at increased risk of developing various viral and bacterial infections. They should be immunized against pneumococcus, meningococcus, mumps, measles, rubella, diphtheria, tetanus and varicella zoster virus. They are also prone to develop osteopenia, osteoporosis and deficiency of iron, vitamin and micronutrients. Baseline bone densitometry should be done, and calcium, vitamin D, iron, vitamin B12, folic acid and fat-soluble vitamins supplementation should be considered. Patients with Crohn's disease are also at risk of developing of skin cancer (melanoma and non-melanoma). Thiopurines increase the chance of developing non-melanoma skin cancer and there is an increased risk of developing melanoma after using biologic agents (anti-TNF, anti-integrin). Patients should avoid sun exposure by using sunscreens and annual skin cancer surveillance should be done by the dermatologist. Patients with perianal Crohn's disease are at increased risk of developing Human Papilloma Virus (HPV)-related anal canal squamous cell cancer and very rarely anal canal adenocarcinoma. They should receive HPV vaccination to reduce HPV-related malignancy. Female patients with Crohn's disease on immunomodulators or biologic agents have increased risk of developing cervical high-grade dysplasia/cancer. They should have regular PAP smear to prevent cervical neoplasia. Female patients with Crohn's disease in remission have the same chance of having conception, normal pregnancy and delivery as normal women without Crohn's disease. Pregnancy can have beneficial effects on Crohn's disease such as less symptoms during pregnancy, less future flare up and less need of future surgery. But if the disease is active, the chance of becoming pregnant is much less. Active disease during pregnancy can cause miscarriage, premature delivery and stillbirth. Thiopurines and anti-TNF agents are safe to be used throughout the pregnancy, and breastfeeding is also compatible with both agents. Methotrexate is teratogenic and cannot be used during pregnancy or lactation. In fact, both man and woman should stop taking MTX 3 months prior to planned pregnancy [5].

Taking care of mental health is another important part of management of Crohn's disease. Patients may suffer from anxiety, depression and narcotic related problems. Various factors may contribute to psychiatric comorbidity which include pain, insomnia, psychosocial stress, frequent hospitalizations, surgical procedures, presence of ostomy, history of proctocolectomy, long duration of Crohn's disease and history of traumatic childhood experiences [6]. During each outpatient visit, patients should be asked about their mental and emotional wellbeing, and appropriate referral to the psychologist or psychiatrist should be given.

In conclusion, Crohn's disease is primarily an idiopathic chronic inflammatory bowel disease with the potential of involving multiple organs. Benign and malignant complications as well as psychiatric comorbidity can occur. Management of Crohn's disease may require multi-specialty team that include primary care physician, gastroenterologist, surgeon, dietitian, interventional radiologist, obstetrician, gynecologist, oncologist, dermatologist, psychiatrist and psychologist. Preventive healthcare and mental healthcare are also very important part of management of Crohn's disease. There are many support groups available in national organizations in individual countries such as Crohn's and Colitis Foundation of America, National Association for Colitis and Crohn's Disease in the United Kingdom, and Crohn's and Colitis Australia. Patients with Crohn's disease should join these support groups where they can communicate, find emotional supports, get answers to their questions and share their experiences with others living with the same disease.

Author details

Monjur Ahmed
Thomas Jefferson University, Philadelphia, Pennsylvania, USA

*Address all correspondence to: monjur.ahmed@jefferson.edu

References

[1] Molodecky NA, Soon IS, Rabi DM, Ghali WA, Ferris M, Chernoff G, Benchimol EI, Panaccione R, Ghosh S, Barkema HW, Kaplan GG. Increasing incidence and prevalence of the inflammatory bowel diseases with time, based on systematic review. Gastroenterology. 2012 Jan; 142(1): 46-54.e42; quiz e30. doi: 10.1053/j.gastro.2011.10.001. Epub 2011 Oct 14. PMID: 22001864.

[2] Kochar B, Barnes EL, Herfarth HH, Martin CF, Ananthakrishnan AN, McGovern D, Long M, Sandler RS. Asians have more perianal Crohn disease and ocular manifestations compared with white Americans. Inflamm Intest Dis. 2018 Mar;2(3): 147-153. doi: 10.1159/000484347. Epub 2017 Nov 18. PMID: 29876356; PMCID: PMC5986188.

[3] Kopylov U, Ben-Horin S, Seidman E. Therapeutic drug monitoring in inflammatory bowel disease. Ann Gastroenterol. 2014;27(4):304-312. PMID: 25331715; PMCID: PMC4188926.

[4] Dittrich AE, Sutton RT, Haynes K, Wang H, Fedorak RN, Kroeker KI. Incidence Rates for Surgery in Crohn's Disease Have Decreased: A Population-based Time-trend Analysis. Inflamm Bowel Dis. 2020 Nov 19;26(12):1909-1916. doi: 10.1093/ibd/izz315. PMID: 31895949.

[5] Puchner A, Gröchenig HP, Sautner J, Helmy-Bader Y, Juch H, Reinisch S, Högenauer C, Koch R, Hermann J, Studnicka-Benke A, Weger W, Puchner R, Dejaco C. Immunosuppressives and biologics during pregnancy and lactation : A consensus report issued by the Austrian Societies of Gastroenterology and Hepatology and Rheumatology and Rehabilitation. Wien Klin Wochenschr. 2019 Jan;131(1-2):29-44. doi: 10.1007/s00508-019-1448-y. Epub 2019 Jan 14. PMID: 30643992; PMCID: PMC6342891.

[6] Schwartz RA, Schwartz IK. Psychiatric disorders associated with Crohn's disease. Int J Psychiatry Med. 1982;12(1):67-73. doi: 10.2190/fl8y-1wu6-1n5l-1fqv. PMID: 7095983.

Chapter 2

Extra-Intestinal Features of Crohn's Disease

Monjur Ahmed

Abstract

Although Crohn's disease is a chronic inflammatory disease of the gastrointestinal tract, it can affect multiple organs behaving like a multisystem immune mediated disease. The dysregulated immune system in patients with Crohn's disease leads to uncontrolled inflammation which primarily affects the gastrointestinal tract but may also affect various extra-intestinal organs. With the increased incidence and prevalence of Crohn's disease, its extra-intestinal manifestations are increasingly being seen in our clinical practice. The musculoskeletal, mucocutaneous, ophthalmic, hepatobiliary, renal, cardiovascular and pulmonary manifestations of Crohn's disease have been reviewed in this chapter. Some of these extra-intestinal manifestations are due to systemic inflammation, some of them are due to malabsorption of nutrients and bile salts, and some due to medications given for the treatment of Crohn's disease. These extra-intestinal manifestations of Crohn's disease are seen in at least 25% of patients with Crohn's disease. Some of them correlate well with Crohn's disease activity but the rest of them have no relation to the activity of Crohn's disease. Although most of the time the extra-intestinal features are seen after the diagnosis of Crohn's disease, they can precede or follow the diagnosis of Crohn's disease. Management of these extra-intestinal manifestations varies as the ones associated with activity of Crohn's disease respond to remission of Crohn's disease whereas the ones not related to the activity of Crohn's disease require specific treatments for those conditions.

Keywords: extra-intestinal manifestations of Crohn's disease, musculoskeletal manifestations of Crohn's disease, mucocutaneous manifestations of Crohn's disease, ophthalmic manifestations of Crohn's disease, hepatobiliary, renal, cardiovascular and pulmonary manifestations of Crohn's disease

1. Introduction

Crohn's disease is an idiopathic chronic, relapsing inflammatory condition that mainly affects the gastrointestinal tract but can also involve extra-intestinal sites. As the incidence and prevalence of this disease is increasing, we are also seeing more and more extra-intestinal features of this disease [1, 2]. Crohn's disease and ulcerative colitis are the two main forms of inflammatory bowel diseases and both of them have extra-intestinal manifestations. In this chapter, we will be focusing on the extra-intestinal features of Crohn's disease.

The gastrointestinal tract plays an important role in immune regulation. The innate and adaptive immunity becomes dysregulated in Crohn's disease. This generally occurs in a genetically susceptible individual due to environmental factors and altered gut microbiota. As the immune homeostasis is disrupted, uncontrolled inflammation occurs in the gut. The inflammatory process can become systemic and other organs can be involved as well. At least 25% of patients with Crohn's disease develop extra-intestinal manifestations [3]. Joints, bones and skin are most commonly involved. Other organs of involvement include muscles, eyes, oral mucosa, hepatobiliary system, kidneys and lungs [4]. Some of these manifestations correlate with disease activity and some of them have no correlation with disease activity. Most of the time joint, eye and skin involvement correlate with intestinal inflammatory disease activity. Active Crohn's disease can reduce fertility in women due to decreased ovarian reserve. This results in decreased anti-Mullerian hormone (AMH) level in the blood in women above age 30 years with active Crohn's colitis compared to healthy control women [5]. Patients' with Crohn's disease have significantly increased risk of developing anxiety and depression, particularly in the year after the initial diagnosis of Crohn's disease [6]. The pooled prevalence of anxiety and depression in Crohn's disease was found to be 31% and 24.4% respectively in a systematic review [7]. Extra-intestinal manifestations (EIMs) are more prevalent in patients with Crohn's colitis although these manifestations may precede the development of colitis, be synchronous with colitis, follow the diagnosis of Crohn's disease or persist even after colitis subsides. Patients with one EIM are at increased risk of developing another EIM. In fact, 25% of the patients have more than one EIM.

2. Musculoskeletal manifestations

As mentioned before musculoskeletal system involvement is common and these include arthalgia, arthritis, pseudoarthritis, hypertrophic osteoarthropathy, osteopenia, osteoporosis, aseptic necrosis of the hip and other joints, psoas abscess, osteomyelitis and sarcopenia. Peripheral arthalgia occurs in about 20% of patients with Crohn's disease and is strongly associated with Crohn's colitis [8]. About 15 to 20% patients with Crohn's disease develop arthritis [9]. Approximately 60 to 70% of arthritis is peripheral large joint arthritis. Knees, ankles, wrists, elbows and hips are most commonly affected. Oligoarticular arthritis affecting less than 5 joints is seen in 6% of patients with Crohn's disease, and polyarticular arthritis affecting 5 or more joints affects 4% of patients with Crohn's disease [10]. A minority of patients with Crohn's disease may develop symmetrical polyarthritis affecting proximal interphalangeal, metacarpophalangeal, and metatarsophalangeal joints similar to the presentation of rheumatoid arthritis. 1 to 6% of patients with Crohn's disease develop ankolysing spondylitis affecting the spine and sacroiliac joints. Patients with ankolysing spondylitis present with low back pain and gradually they develop spinal fusion over a period of time. As many as two-third of patients with Crohn's disease with ankolysing spondylitis are HLA-B27 positive [11]. Small joint polyarthritis and ankolysing spondylitis can flare up without any increased activity of Crohn's disease. Pseudoarthritis presenting as diffuse joint aches can occur following glucocorticoids withdrawal. Aseptic necrosis of joints (particularly hip joints) can occur in Crohn's disease due to hypercoagulable state and fibrin microclot formation occluding the epiphyseal capillaries [12]. Either short term high dose or long term corticosteroid therapy can also predispose the patients with Crohn's disease to aseptic necrosis of bone (i.e. cellular death of bone) which can cause severe pain and disability [13]. In one study, 2.1% of patients with inflammatory bowel disease had aseptic necrosis of the hip on computerized tomography [14]. Crohn's disease leads to low mineral density which is seen even at time of diagnosis. Proinflammatory cytokines like tumor necrosis factor, smoking, calcium and vitamin D malabsorption and low body mass index (BMI) are contributing factors although use of glucocorticoids is the main risk factor [15, 16]. Osteopenia (T score − 1.0 to −2.49) and osteoporosis (T score − 2.5 and lower) are seen in 30 to 60% of patients with Crohn's disease. 60% of patients with Crohn's disease also develop sarcopenia that is strongly related to osteopenia and osteoporosis [17].

In a nutshell, the various manifestations are as follows:

- Arthritis
  - a. Large joint
    - 1. Polyarticular
    - 2. Oligoaticular
  - b. Symmetrical small joint
  - c. Ankolysing spondylitis
- Peripheral arthlagia
- Pseudoarhritis
- Hypertrophic osteoarthropathy
- Osteopenia, osteoporosis
- Sarcopenia
- Aseptic necrosis of the hip and other joints
- Psoas abscess
- Osteomyelitis

3. Mucocutaneous manifestations

Cutaneous manifestations occur in almost one third of patients with Crohn's disease. Erythema nodosum (EN) and pyoderma gangrenosum (PG) are the most common cutaneous lesions seen in Crohn's disease although these lesions can also be seen in other disorders [18]. EN appears as an erythematous subcutaneous tender nodule, most commonly seen on the pretibial region (**Figure 1**). In Crohn's disease, EN is more commonly seen in females than in males. It tends to occur during the first 2 years of clinical course and is associated with exacerbation of large joint arthritis and colitis, and generally improves with the treatment of Crohn's disease [19]. It is recommended not to biopsy EN because of risk of scar tissue formation.

PG generally presents as painful ulcers with sharply circumscribed and demarcated violacious borders and crater-like holes at the necrotic yellowish base, most commonly seen on the extensor surface of the lower extremities but can occur anywhere on the body [20]. Sometimes PG can present tender nodules or pustules [21]. PG is a chronic debilitating skin disorder and is not associated with Crohn's

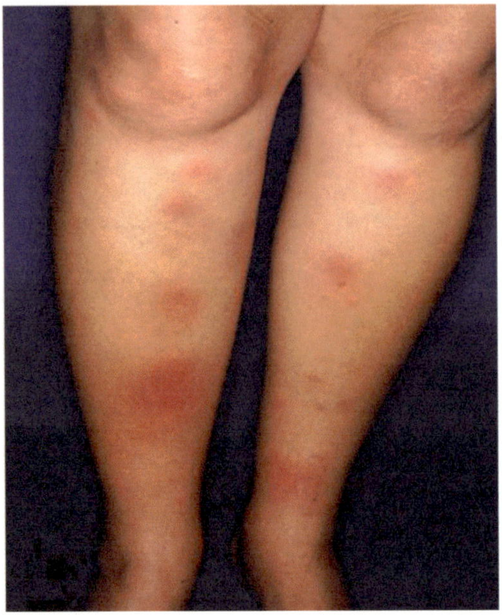

Figure 1.
Erythema nodusum.

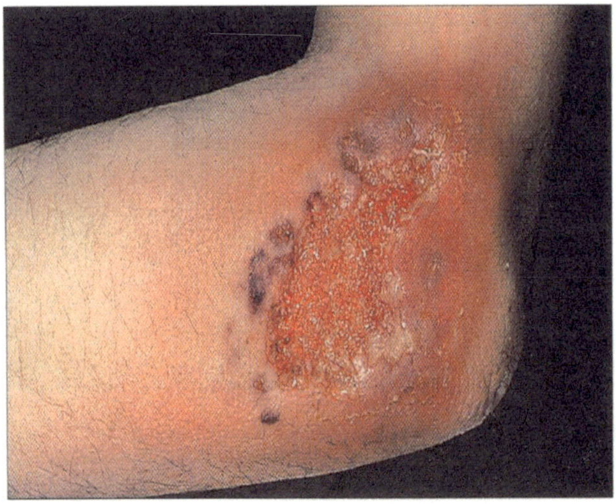

Figure 2.
Pyoderma gangrenosum.

disease activity. Histologically it is a neutrophilic dermatosis characterized by infiltration of neutrophils into the skin. Pathergy phenomenon (i.e. formation of large ulcers in response to minor trauma) is characteristic of PG. PG heals up with cribriform scars (**Figure 2**).

Sweet's syndrome (SS) is another neutrophilic dermatosis rarely associated with Crohn's disease. Patients present with painful erythematous or violaceous papular or nodular lesions on the face, neck or upper extremity with abrupt onset of fever and neutrophlic leukocytosis [22].

Oral mucosa can be affected in Crohn's disease. Lips are the most common sites of oral Crohn's disease [23]. Lips become swollen with vertical fissures due to granulomatous involvement of the lips. Aphthous ulcers or stomatitis (AS) occurs in 20 to 30% of patients with Crohn's disease [24]. Pyostomatitis vegetans (PV) is another rare lesion associated with Crohn's disease. It is characterized by 'snail track' shaped flat yellowish ulcers in the oral and gingival mucosa [25].

Another rare cutaneous manifestation of Crohn's disease is metastatic Crohn's disease (MCD). It can present as papule, nodule, plaque or ulcer with a predilection for skin folds, external genitalia (penis, vulva), perineum, infra-mammary area, limbs and retroauricular area [26]. It is so called because of the presence of non-caseating granuloma (histologically identical to the primary intestinal lesion) in the skin that is remote from the gastrointestinal tract [27]. MCD can precede or develop simultaneously with intestinal Crohn's disease. No clear correlation is found between MCD and intestinal Crohn's disease activity [28].

The prevalence of psoriasis is 8 times higher in patients with Crohn's disease than that in the general population due to overlapping genetic and immunopathogenic mechanisms [29]. There is also increased incidence of epidermolysis bullosa acquisita and leucocytoclastic vasculitis in patients with Crohn's disease [30, 31]. Epidermolysis bullosa acquisita (EBA) appears as subepidermal blistering skin lesion over the extensor aspect of the body, particularly on trauma prone areas, and is associated with scarring, milia formation and skin fragility. EBA occurs due to autoimmunity to type VII collagen present at the dermoepidermal junction and is associated with symptomatic esophageal web formation [32]. Leucocytoclastic vasculitis (LCV) is another very rare dermatologic manifestation of Crohn's disease and presents as palpable purpura over the lower extremities and ankles [33]. EN, AS, PV, SS and LCV can be associated with increased intestinal inflammatory activity.

Dermatologic manifestations secondary to malabsorption of nutrients can occur. These include angular cheilitis due to riboflavin deficiency, purpura due to vitamin K deficiency and acrodermatitis enteropathica (AE) due to zinc deficiency. AE appears as eczematoid and psoriasiform patchy skin lesions on the extremities and peri-orificially. AE can also cause alopecia [34].

Patients with Crohn's disease are at increased risk of developing melanoma of the skin [35].

Certain skin lesions are due to the medications used to control Crohn's disease. Anti-tumor necrosis factor (TNF) agents can cause paradoxical psoriasiform rash over the palmar aspect of hands, planter aspects of feet, flexures and scalp in about 5% of patients [36]. Risk factors for developing this rash include female sex, obesity, smoking (active or past), short duration of disease and family history of inflammatory skin disease [37]. The pathogenesis of development of this anti-TNF-induced psoriasiform rash is exactly not known. But increased concentration of IL-17/IL-22 expressing Th17 cells and interferon (IFN)- ϒ-expressing Th1 cells are seen in the rash [36, 38]. IFN- α may also play a role in the formation of this rash. Normally TNF decreases the production of IFN- α by inhibiting the maturation of plasmacytoid dendritic cells. Anti-TNF therapy may lead to overproduction of IFN-α [39]. Increased concentration of IFN- α protein is found in anti-TNF associated psoriasiform rash. Another mechanism could be anti-TNF-induced patchy cutaneous immune suppression leading to the formation of psoriasiform rash [40].

Other non-psoriasiform skin lesions due to anti-TNF agents include local pruritic skin erythema at the site of infusion, eczematiform skin lesions, xerosis cutis, palmoplantar pustulosis, viral and bacterial infections of the skin [41]. Long et all found in a retrospective study that ant-TNF therapy may increase the risk of melanoma, and thiopurines may increase the risk of non-melanoma skin cancer (basal cell cancer, squamous cell cancer) [42]. The mucocutaneous manifestations are outlined in **Table 1**.

Mucocutaneous manifestations due to disease	Mucocutaneous manifestations due to malabsorption	Mucocutaneous manifestations due to medications
• Erythema nodosum • Pyoderma gangrenosum • Sweet's syndrome • Aphthous ulcers or stomatitis • Pyostomatitis vegetans • Granulomatous cheilitis • Metastatic Crohn's disease • Epidermolysis bullosa acquisita • Leucocytoclastic vasculitis • increased risk of developing melanoma of the skin	• angular cheilitis • Purpura • Acrodermatitis enteropathica	• Paradoxical psoriasiform rash due to anti-TNF • local pruritic skin erythema at the site of infusion • Eczematiform skin lesions • Xerosis cutis • Palmoplantar pustulosis • Viral and bacterial infections of the skin • Increased risk of melanoma due to anti-TNF • Increased risk of non-melanoma skin cancer (basal cell cancer, squamous cell cancer) due to thiopurines

Table 1.
Mucocutaneous manifestations of Crohn's disease.

4. Ophthalmic manifestations

Eyes can be involved in 12% of patients with Crohn's disease [43]. Ocular involvement occurs more commonly in patients with colonic or ileocolonic Crohn's disease than in patients with isolated small bowel Crohn's disease [44]. Frequently, patients with ocular involvement also have peripheral large joint arthritis and EN. The common ophthalmic manifestations include episcleritis, scleritis, uveitis, non-specific follicular conjunctivitis and blepharitis [45]. Rarely, orbital myositis and optic neuritis can occur. Patients with episcleritis and scleritis present with red tender eyes. Patients with uveitis present with deep eye pain, red eyes with circumcorneal congestion, meiosis, headache, blurring of vision and photophobia. Patients with uveitis should be seen by an ophthalmologist emergently. Uveitis in patients with Crohn's disease is generally bilateral, posterior, insidious in onset, chronic and 4 times more common in females than in males [46]. Patients with small bowel Crohn's disease may also present with night blindness secondary to vitamin A malabsorption and deficiency. The ophthalmic manifestations are outlined in **Table 2**.

Ophthalmic manifestations due to disease	Ophthalmic manifestations due to malabsorption
• Episcleritis (**Figure 3**) • Scleritis • Uveitis • Follicular conjunctivitis • Blepharitis • Orbital myositis • Optic neuritis	Night blindness due to vitamin A deficiency

Table 2.
Ophthalmic manifestations in Crohn's disease.

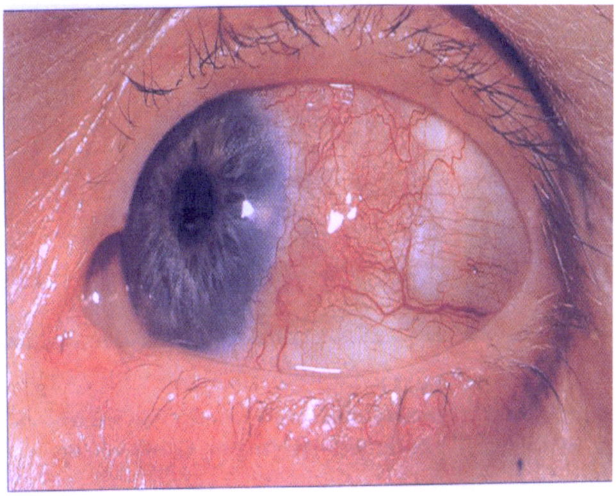

Figure 3.
Episcleritis.

5. Hepatobiliary manifestations

Crohn's disease can affect both liver and biliary tract. Some of the manifestations are directly related to the disease process and some are secondary to medications used in Crohn's disease. Non-alcoholic hepatic steatosis (NAHS) is the most frequent hepatobiliary manifestation that is secondary to intestinal inflammation and metabolic factors [47]. Sagami et all found in a retrospective study that patients with Crohn's disease and NAHS had higher rate of remission and longer surgery free interval [48]. About 2% of patients with Crohn's disease develop primary sclerosing cholangitis (PSC), and 5 to 10% of patients with PSC have Crohn's disease [49]. PSC is a progressive inflammatory, fibrosing and stricturing disease involving both intrahepatic and extrahepatic bile ducts in more than 80% of cases. In about 10% of cases, only intrahepatic bile ducts are involved and in less than 5% of cases, only extrahepatic bile ducts are involved. Patients with PSC remain asymptomatic for many years. They are generally detected by finding abnormal liver function test. When symptomatic, they generally present with itching jaundice, right upper quadrant pain, fever and chills. Magnatic resonance cholangiopancreatography (MRCP) rather than Endoscopic retrograde cholangiopancreatography (ERCP) is now considered as diagnostic test of choice as it is non-invasive, can reduce the risk of hospitalization by 10%, and can visualize the liver [50]. It shows 'stricturing and beading' appearance of both extra-hepatic and intra-hepatic bile ducts. Liver biopsy is not required if imaging studies are suggestive of PSC. Liver histology may show lymphocytic infiltrate of bile duct, bile ductopenia, and periductal concentric fibrosis giving 'onion skin' appearance but no histological appearance is pathognomonic of PSC. Patients with PSC are at increased (10–15%) risk of developing cholangiocarcinoma. But colon cancer risk does not seem to be increased in patients with PSC and Crohn's colitis [51]. Other hepatobiliary manifestations of Crohn's disease include cholelithiasis, granulomatous hepatitis, portal vein thrombosis and secondary amyloidosis [52–54]. Patients with Crohn's disease have 2 fold increased prevalence of gallstone formation than general population. According to Crohn's and colitis foundation of America, up to one third of patients with Crohn's disease may develop gallstones which could be cholesterol-rich stones or pigment stones. In Crohn's disease, gallbladder bile may get supersatuarated with cholesterol (with or

Renal manifestations due to disease	Renal manifestations due to malabsorption	Renal manifestations due to medications
• IgA nephropathy • Membranous glomeruloneohritis • Tubulointerstitial nephritis • Amyloidosis	• Nephrolithiasis	• Interstitial nephritis

Table 3.
Renal manifestations in Crohn's disease.

without ileal disease/resection) leading to the formation of cholesterol-rich gallstones [55]. In patients with ileal disease/resection, bile acid malabsorption initially causes bile acid-induced diarrhea. Bile acid pool slowly decreases and it leads to cholesterol supersaturated bile and cholesterol-rich stone formation. Bile acid malabsorption also induces enterohepatic circulation of bilirubin and increases the rate of secretion of bilirubin into bile. This may help formation of pigment stone [56].

6. Renal manifestations

Renal and urinary tract involvement can occur rarely in Crohn's disease. Nephrolithiasis, IgA nephropathy, membranous glomeruloneohritis, tubulointerstitial nephritis and amyloidosis are the most frequent involvement [57]. Calcium oxalate stone is formed in the kidneys and urinary tract because of hyperoxaluria. In extensive Crohn's disease of small bowel or intestinal resection, malabsorbed free fatty acid binds calcium in the intestinal lumen to form calcium-fatty acid salts and thus free calcium becomes less available to bind oxalate in the intestinal lumen. Oxalate then binds with sodium to form sodium oxalate that is easily absorbed through the colonic mucosa resulting in hyperoxaluria [58]. Uric acid stones can also be formed in patients with diarrhea and/or intestinal neostomy, dehydration and hypemetabolic state [59]. Crohn's disease is also associated with IgA nephropathy [60] and membranous glomerulonephritis [61]. Patients taking mesalamine can develop interstitial nephritis. But patients with Crohn's disease (not taking mesalamine) can also develop primary chronic tubulointerstitial nephritis [62]. Secondary renal amyloidosis can be a late manifestation of Crohn's disease [63]. The renal manifestations are outlined in **Table 3**.

7. Cardiovascular manifestations

Although different cardiovascular manifestations are seen in patients with Crohn's disease, they are not due to traditional cardiovascular risk factors but secondary to chronic systemic inflammation [64]. The different cardiovascular manifestations include pericarditis, myocarditis, nonbacterial thrombotic endocarditis, congestive heart failure, arterial and venous thromboembolism. Among these pericarditis is the most common cardiovascular manifestation [65]. Myocarditis can be due to autoimmune mechanism secondary to exposure to autoantigen or mesalamine-induced [66]. Crohn's disease can also be associated with non-bacterial thrombotic endocarditis (Libman-Sacks endocarditis) due to hypercoagulable state [67]. The chronic inflammatory state seen in Crohn's disease may cause myocardial fibrosis due to abnormal collagen metabolism, microvascular endothelial dysfunction, vitamin and essential nutrient deficiencies and changes in nitric oxide mediated vasodilation [68]. This may lead to chronic heart failure, atrial and ventricular arrhythmia and heart block. Acute heart failure can occur secondary to myopericarditis or myocardial infarction. Patients with Crohn's disease are at increased risk of developing both venous and arterial thromoboembolism because of hypercoagulable state as active bowel inflammation leads to thrombocytosis, increased levels of factor V, factor VIII, fibrinogen and fibrinopeptide A, and deficiency of antithrombin III and free protein S in the blood. Other factors include prolonged bed rest, immobility, central venous catheter placement, use of corticosteroids and oral contraceptive pills, smoking and dehydration [69]. The cardiovascular manifestations are outlined as follows:

- Pericarditis
- Myocarditis
- Nonbacterial thrombotic endocarditis
- Increased risk of thromboembolism

8. Pulmonary manifestations

Patients with Crohn's disease can rarely develop subclinical inflammatory process in the lung parenchyma, tracheobronchial tree and pleura in the absence of pulmonary symptoms [70, 71]. Increased lymphocytic count in bronchoalveolar lavage (BAL) indicating lymphocytic alveolitis may suggest latent involvement of lungs in Crohn's disease [72]. Abnormal pulmonary function test (increased carbon monoxide transfer factor/TLCO) can be found in this asymptomatic group of patients without any abnormal imaging [73]. Lung involvement may correlate with bowel inflammation [74]. Other pulmonary manifestations seen in association with Crohn's disease are tracheobronchitis, bronchiectasis, bronchiolitis obliterans organizing pneumonia (BOOP), multiple pulmonary nodules (sterile necrobiotic nodules consisting of sterile aggregates of neutrophils with necrosis), pleuropericarditis, methotrexate-induced pneumonitis, interstitial lung disease and pulmonary eosinophilia due to sulfasalazine and mesalamine, and biologic agents related infections such as reactivation of pulmonary tuberculosis, development of pneumocystis carinii pneumonia and opportunistic fungal infections (aspergillosis, coccidiomycosis, histoplasmosis, nocardiosis) [75–84]. The pulmonary manifestations are outlined in **Table 4**.

Pulmonary manifestations due to disease	Pulmonary manifestations due to medications
• Lymphocytic alveolitis • Tracheobronchitis • Bronchiectasis • Bronchiolitis obliterans organizing pneumonia • Multiple pulmonary nodules • Pleuropericarditis	• Methotrexate-induced pneumonitis and interstitial lung disease • Pulmonary eosinophilia due to sulfasalazine and mesalamine • Reactivation of pulmonary tuberculosis, development of pneumocystis carinii pneumonia and opportunistic fungal infections (aspergillosis, coccidiomycosis, histoplasmosis, nocardiosis) due biologic agents

Table 4.
Pulmonary manifestations in Crohn's disease.

9. Conclusion

As Crohn's disease is a chronic systemic inflammatory disease, the inflammatory cascade can be seen in multiple organs. Many of the EIMs occur as a result of pro-inflammatory cytokines. Some of the EIMs do not correlate with intestinal inflammatory activity. Some of the EIMs may precede the gastrointestinal manifestations of Crohn's disease. Some of the EIMs are due to malabsorption of nutrients, vitamins and minerals. Some of the EIMs are due to autoantigens. Some of the EIMs are due to medications used for Crohn's disease.

Author details

Monjur Ahmed
Thomas Jefferson University, Philadelphia, Pennsylvania, USA

*Address all correspondence to: monjur.ahmed@jefferson.edu

References

[1] Torres J, Mehandru S, Colombel JF, Peyrin-Biroulet L. Crohn's disease. Lancet. 2017 Apr 29; 389(10080): 1741-1755. doi: 10.1016/S0140-6736(16) 31711-1. Epub 2016 Dec 1. PMID: 27914655.

[2] Veauthier B, Hornecker JR. Crohn's Disease: Diagnosis and Management. Am Fam Physician. 2018 Dec 1;98(11): 661-669. PMID: 30485038.

[3] Ephgrave K. Extra-intestinal manifestations of Crohn's disease. Surg Clin North Am. 2007 Jun;87(3):673-680. doi: 10.1016/j.suc.2007.03.003. PMID: 17560419.

[4] Levine JS, Burakoff R. Extraintestinal manifestations of inflammatory bowel disease. Gastroenterol Hepatol (N Y). 2011 Apr;7(4):235-41. PMID: 21857821; PMCID: PMC3127025.

[5] Fréour T, Miossec C, Bach-Ngohou K, Dejoie T, Flamant M, Maillard O, Denis MG, Barriere P, Bruley des Varannes S, Bourreille A, Masson D. Ovarian reserve in young women of reproductive age with Crohn's disease. Inflamm Bowel Dis. 2012 Aug;18(8): 1515-1522. doi: 10.1002/ibd.21872. Epub 2011 Sep 20. PMID: 21936034.

[6] Kurina LM, Goldacre MJ, Yeates D, Gill LE. Depression and anxiety in people with inflammatory bowel disease. J Epidemiol Community Health. 2001 Oct;55(10):716-20. doi: 10.1136/ jech.55.10.716. PMID: 11553654; PMCID: PMC1731788.

[7] Mikocka-Walus A, Knowles SR, Keefer L, Graff L. Controversies Revisited: A Systematic Review of the Comorbidity of Depression and Anxiety with Inflammatory Bowel Diseases. Inflamm Bowel Dis. 2016 Mar;22(3): 752-762. doi: 10.1097/ MIB.0000000000000620. PMID: 26841224.

[8] Farmer RG, Hawk WA, Turnbull RB Jr. Clinical patterns in Crohn's disease: a statistical study of 615 cases. Gastroenterology. 1975 Apr;68(4 Pt 1): 627-635. PMID: 1123132.

[9] Orchard TR. Management of arthritis in patients with inflammatory bowel disease. Gastroenterol Hepatol (N Y). 2012 May;8(5):327-9. PMID: 22933865; PMCID: PMC3424429.

[10] Orchard TR, Wordsworth BP, Jewell DP. Peripheral arthropathies in inflammatory bowel disease: their articular distribution and natural history. Gut. 1998 Mar;42(3):387-91. doi: 10.1136/gut.42.3.387. PMID: 9577346; PMCID: PMC1727027.

[11] Jacques P, Mielants H, Coppieters K, De Vos M, Elewaut D. The intimate relationship between gut and joint in spondyloarthropathies. Curr Opin Rheumatol. 2007 Jul;19(4):353-357. doi: 10.1097/BOR.0b013e328133f59f. PMID: 17551365.

[12] Khan A, Illiffe G, Houston DS, Bernstein CN. Osteonecrosis in a patient with Crohn's disease unrelated to corticosteroid use. Can J Gastroenterol. 2001 Nov;15(11):765-768. doi: 10.1155/ 2001/293059. PMID: 11727007.

[13] Klingenstein G, Levy RN, Kornbluth A, Shah AK, Present DH. Inflammatory bowel disease related osteonecrosis: report of a large series with a review of the literature. Aliment Pharmacol Ther. 2005 Feb 1;21(3): 243-249. doi: 10.1111/ j.1365-2036.2005.02231.x. PMID: 15691298.

[14] Rolston VS, Patel AV, Learch TJ, Li D, Karayev D, Williams C, Siddanthi ML, Targan SR, Weisman MH, McGovern DPB. Prevalence and Associations of Avascular Necrosis of the Hip in a Large

Well-characterized Cohort of Patients With Inflammatory Bowel Disease. J Clin Rheumatol. 2019 Jan;25(1):45-49. doi: 10.1097/RHU.0000000000000797. PMID: 29794876; PMCID: PMC6252167.

[15] Turk N, Cukovic-Cavka S, Korsic M, Turk Z, Vucelic B. Proinflammatory cytokines and receptor activator of nuclear factor kappaB-ligand/ osteoprotegerin associated with bone deterioration in patients with Crohn's disease. Eur J Gastroenterol Hepatol. 2009 Feb;21(2):159-166. doi: 10.1097/ MEG.0b013e3283200032. PMID: 19098682.

[16] Noble CL, McCullough J, Ho W, Lees CW, Nimmo E, Drummond H, Bear S, Hannan J, Millar C, Ralston SH, Satsangi J. Low body mass not vitamin D receptor polymorphisms predict osteoporosis in patients with inflammatory bowel disease. Aliment Pharmacol Ther. 2008 Apr 1;27(7): 588-596. doi: 10.1111/ j.1365-2036.2008.03599.x. Epub 2008 Jan 10. PMID: 18194505.

[17] Schneider SM, Al-Jaouni R, Filippi J, Wiroth JB, Zeanandin G, Arab K, Hébuterne X. Sarcopenia is prevalent in patients with Crohn's disease in clinical remission. Inflamm Bowel Dis. 2008 Nov;14(11):1562-1568. doi: 10.1002/ ibd.20504. PMID: 18478564.

[18] Lebwohl M, Lebwohl O. Cutaneous manifestations of inflammatory bowel disease. Inflamm Bowel Dis. 1998 May;4 (2):142-148. doi: 10.1002/ ibd.3780040209. PMID: 9589299.

[19] Tavarela Veloso F. Review article: skin complications associated with inflammatory bowel disease. Aliment Pharmacol Ther. 2004 Oct;20 Suppl 4: 50-53. doi: 10.1111/ j.1365-2036.2004.02055.x. PMID: 15352894.

[20] Yeh JE, Tsiaras WG. Intractable pyoderma gangrenosum in a Crohn's disease patient on vedolizumab. JAAD Case Rep. 2017 Mar 9;3(2):110-112. doi: 10.1016/j.jdcr.2017.01.012. PMID: 28337471; PMCID: PMC5347515.

[21] Brooklyn T, Dunnill G, Probert C. Diagnosis and treatment of pyoderma gangrenosum. BMJ. 2006 Jul 22;333 (7560):181-4. doi: 10.1136/ bmj.333.7560.181. PMID: 16858047; PMCID: PMC1513476.

[22] Lima CDS, Pinto RDB, Góes HFO, Salles SAN, Vilar EAG, Lima CDS. Sweet's syndrome associated with Crohn's disease. An Bras Dermatol. 2017 Mar-Apr;92(2):263-265. doi: 10.1590/ abd1806-4841.20175298. PMID: 28538894; PMCID: PMC5429120.

[23] Plauth M, Jenss H, Meyle J. Oral manifestations of Crohn's disease. An analysis of 79 cases. J Clin Gastroenterol. 1991 Feb;13(1):29-37. doi: 10.1097/ 00004836-199102000-00008. PMID: 2007740.

[24] Trikudanathan G, Venkatesh PG, Navaneethan U. Diagnosis and therapeutic management of extra-intestinal manifestations of inflammatory bowel disease. Drugs. 2012 Dec 24;72(18):2333-2349. doi: 10.2165/11638120-000000000-00000. PMID: 23181971.

[25] Huang BL, Chandra S, Shih DQ. Skin manifestations of inflammatory bowel disease. Front Physiol. 2012 Feb 6;3:13. doi: 10.3389/fphys.2012.00013. PMID: 22347192; PMCID: PMC3273725.

[26] Panackel C, John J, Krishnadas D, Vinayakumar KR. Metastatic Crohn's disease of external genitalia. Indian J Dermatol. 2008;53(3):146-8. doi: 10.4103/0019-5154.43207. PMID: 19882017; PMCID: PMC2763745.

[27] Palamaras I, El-Jabbour J, Pietropaolo N, Thomson P, Mann S, Robles W, Stevens HP. Metastatic Crohn's disease: a review. J Eur Acad

Dermatol Venereol. 2008 Sep;22(9): 1033-1043. doi: 10.1111/ j.1468-3083.2008.02741.x. Epub 2008 Jun 19. PMID: 18573158.

[28] Graham DB, Jager DL, Borum ML. Metastatic Crohn's disease of the face. Dig Dis Sci. 2006 Nov;51(11):2062-2063. doi: 10.1007/s10620-006-9533-2. Epub 2006 Sep 29. PMID: 17009111.

[29] Fiorino G, Omodei PD. Psoriasis and Inflammatory Bowel Disease: Two Sides of the Same Coin? J Crohns Colitis. 2015 Sep;9(9):697-698. doi: 10.1093/ecco-jcc/ jjv110. Epub 2015 Jun 15. PMID: 26079725.

[30] Reddy H, Shipman AR, Wojnarowska F. Epidermolysis bullosa acquisita and inflammatory bowel disease: a review of the literature. Clin Exp Dermatol. 2013 Apr;38(3):225-229; quiz 229-30. doi: 10.1111/ced.12114. PMID: 23517353.

[31] Tsiamoulos Z, Karamanolis G, Polymeros D, Triantafyllou K, Oikonomopoulos T. Leukocytoclastic vasculitis as an onset symptom of Crohn's disease. Case Rep Gastroenterol. 2008 Sep;2(3):410-4. doi: 10.1159/ 000161562. Epub 2008 Nov 14. PMID: 21897791; PMCID: PMC3166803.

[32] Stewart MI, Woodley DT, Briggaman RA. Epidermolysis bullosa acquisita and associated symptomatic esophageal webs. Arch Dermatol. 1991 Mar;127(3):373-377. PMID: 1998368.

[33] Buck M, Dumic I, McDermott W, Nordstrom C, Dawan S, Virata A, Martin S, Hudson A, Milovanovic T, Nordin T. Leukocytoclastic vasculitis as a rare dermatologic manifestation of Crohn's disease mimicking cellulitis: a case report. BMC Gastroenterol. 2020 Jul 29;20(1):240. doi: 10.1186/ s12876-020-01371-3. PMID: 32727390; PMCID: PMC7389435.

[34] Krasovec M, Frenk E. Acrodermatitis enteropathica secondary to Crohn's disease. Dermatology. 1996; 193(4):361-363. doi: 10.1159/ 000246296. PMID: 8993972.

[35] Kappelman MD, Farkas DK, Long MD, Erichsen R, Sandler RS, Sørensen HT, Baron JA. Risk of cancer in patients with inflammatory bowel diseases: a nationwide population-based cohort study with 30 years of follow-up evaluation. Clin Gastroenterol Hepatol. 2014 Feb;12(2):265-73.e1. doi: 10.1016/j. cgh.2013.03.034. Epub 2013 Apr 17. PMID: 23602821; PMCID: PMC4361949.

[36] Cullen G, Kroshinsky D, Cheifetz AS, Korzenik JR. Psoriasis associated with anti-tumour necrosis factor therapy in inflammatory bowel disease: a new series and a review of 120 cases from the literature. Aliment Pharmacol Ther. 2011 Dec;34(11–12):1318-1327. doi: 10.1111/ j.1365-2036.2011.04866.x. Epub 2011 Sep 29. PMID: 21957906.

[37] Tillack C, Ehmann LM, Friedrich M, Laubender RP, Papay P, Vogelsang H, Stallhofer J, Beigel F, Bedynek A, Wetzke M, Maier H, Koburger M, Wagner J, Glas J, Diegelmann J, Koglin S, Dombrowski Y, Schauber J, Wollenberg A, Brand S. Anti-TNF antibody-induced psoriasiform skin lesions in patients with inflammatory bowel disease are characterised by interferon-γ-expressing Th1 cells and IL-17A/IL-22-expressing Th17 cells and respond to anti-IL-12/IL-23 antibody treatment. Gut. 2014 Apr;63(4):567-77. doi: 10.1136/gutjnl-2012-302853. Epub 2013 Mar 6. PMID: 23468464.

[38] Teunissen MB, Koomen CW, de Waal Malefyt R, Wierenga EA, Bos JD. Interleukin-17 and interferon-gamma synergize in the enhancement of proinflammatory cytokine production by human keratinocytes. J Invest Dermatol. 1998 Oct;111(4):645-649. doi: 10.1046/ j.1523-1747.1998.00347.x. PMID: 9764847.

[39] de Gannes GC, Ghoreishi M, Pope J, Russell A, Bell D, Adams S, Shojania K,

Martinka M, Dutz JP. Psoriasis and pustular dermatitis triggered by TNF-{alpha} inhibitors in patients with rheumatologic conditions. Arch Dermatol. 2007 Feb;143(2):223-231. doi: 10.1001/archderm.143.2.223. PMID: 17310002.

[40] Scaldaferri F, Petito V, Papa A, Cesarini M, Arena V, Lopetuso LR, Corbi M, Perino F, Caldarola G, Carbone A, Corazziari E, Sgambato A, Gasbarrini A, De Simone C. Anti-TNF-α-induced psoriasiform lesions in IBD: an abnormal immune activation or a 'patchy cutaneous' immune suppression? Gut. 2014 Apr;63(4): 699-701. doi: 10.1136/gutjnl-2013-305478. Epub 2013 Nov 19. PMID: 24253935.

[41] Cleynen I, Van Moerkercke W, Billiet T, Vandecandelaere P, Vande Casteele N, Breynaert C, Ballet V, Ferrante M, Noman M, Assche GV, Rutgeerts P, van den Oord JJ, Gils A, Segaert S, Vermeire S. Characteristics of Skin Lesions Associated With Anti-Tumor Necrosis Factor Therapy in Patients With Inflammatory Bowel Disease: A Cohort Study. Ann Intern Med. 2016 Jan 5;164(1):10-22. doi: 10.7326/M15-0729. Epub 2015 Dec 8. PMID: 26641955.

[42] Long MD, Martin CF, Pipkin CA, Herfarth HH, Sandler RS, Kappelman MD. Risk of melanoma and nonmelanoma skin cancer among patients with inflammatory bowel disease. Gastroenterology. 2012 Aug;143 (2):390-399.e1. doi: 10.1053/j.gastro.2012.05.004. Epub 2012 May 11. PMID: 22584081; PMCID: PMC4065572.

[43] Kalla R, Ventham NT, Satsangi J, Arnott ID. Crohn's disease. BMJ. 2014 Nov 19;349:g6670. doi: 10.1136/bmj.g6670. PMID: 25409896.

[44] Das KM. Relationship of extraintestinal involvements in inflammatory bowel disease: new insights into autoimmune pathogenesis. Dig Dis Sci. 1999 Jan;44(1):1-13. doi: 10.1023/a:1026629528233. PMID: 9952216.

[45] Mintz R, Feller ER, Bahr RL, Shah SA. Ocular manifestations of inflammatory bowel disease. Inflamm Bowel Dis. 2004 Mar;10(2):135-139. doi: 10.1097/00054725-200403000-00012. PMID: 15168814.

[46] Lyons JL, Rosenbaum JT. Uveitis associated with inflammatory bowel disease compared with uveitis associated with spondyloarthropathy. Arch Ophthalmol. 1997 Jan;115(1): 61-64. doi: 10.1001/archopht.1997.01100150063010. PMID: 9006426.

[47] Magrì S, Paduano D, Chicco F, Cingolani A, Farris C, Delogu G, Tumbarello F, Lai M, Melis A, Casula L, Fantini MC, Usai P. Nonalcoholic fatty liver disease in patients with inflammatory bowel disease: Beyond the natural history. World J Gastroenterol. 2019 Oct 7;25(37):5676-5686. doi: 10.3748/wjg.v25.i37.5676. PMID: 31602167; PMCID: PMC6785525.

[48] Sagami S, Ueno Y, Tanaka S, Fujita A, Hayashi R, Oka S, Hyogo H, Chayama K. Significance of non-alcoholic fatty liver disease in Crohn's disease: A retrospective cohort study. Hepatol Res. 2017 Aug;47(9):872-881. doi: 10.1111/hepr.12828. Epub 2016 Nov 28. PMID: 27737498.

[49] Levine JS, Burakoff R. Extraintestinal manifestations of inflammatory bowel disease. Gastroenterol Hepatol (N Y). 2011 Apr;7 (4):235-41. PMID: 21857821; PMCID: PMC3127025.

[50] Khoshpouri P, Habibabadi RR, Hazhirkarzar B, Ameli S, Ghadimi M, Ghasabeh MA, Menias CO, Kim A, Li Z, Kamel IR. Imaging Features of Primary Sclerosing Cholangitis: From Diagnosis

to Liver Transplant Follow-up. Radiographics. 2019 Nov-Dec;39(7): 1938-1964. doi: 10.1148/rg.2019180213. Epub 2019 Oct 18. PMID: 31626561.

[51] Braden B, Halliday J, Aryasingha S, Sharifi Y, Checchin D, Warren BF, Kitiyakara T, Travis SP, Chapman RW. Risk for colorectal neoplasia in patients with colonic Crohn's disease and concomitant primary sclerosing cholangitis. Clin Gastroenterol Hepatol. 2012 Mar;10(3):303-308. doi: 10.1016/j.cgh.2011.10.020. Epub 2011 Oct 28. PMID: 22037429.

[52] Patedakis Litvinov BI, Pathak AP. Granulomatous hepatitis in a patient with Crohn's disease and cholestasis. BMJ Case Rep. 2017 Sep 7;2017: bcr2017220988. doi: 10.1136/bcr-2017-220988. PMID: 28882937; PMCID: PMC5589046.

[53] Mathieu E, Fain O, Trinchet JC, Aurousseau MH, Stérin D, Thomas M. La thrombose porte: une complication exceptionnelle de la maladie de Crohn [Portal vein thrombosis: a rare complication of Crohn disease]. Rev Med Interne. 1994;15(9):589-92. French. doi: 10.1016/s0248-8663(05)82504-4. PMID: 7984838.

[54] Sharma P, Aguilar R, Siddiqui OA, Nader MA. Secondary systemic amyloidosis in inflammatory bowel disease: a nationwide analysis. Ann Gastroenterol. 2017;30(5):504-511. doi: 10.20524/aog.2017.0168. Epub 2017 Jun 14. PMID: 28845105; PMCID: PMC5566770.

[55] Lapidus A, Akerlund JE, Einarsson C. Gallbladder bile composition in patients with Crohn 's disease. World J Gastroenterol. 2006 Jan 7;12(1):70-4. doi: 10.3748/wjg.v12.i1.70. PMID: 16440420; PMCID: PMC4077498.

[56] Brink MA, Slors JF, Keulemans YC, Mok KS, De Waart DR, Carey MC, Groen AK, Tytgat GN. Enterohepatic cycling of bilirubin: a putative mechanism for pigment gallstone formation in ileal Crohn's disease. Gastroenterology. 1999 Jun;116(6): 1420-1427. doi: 10.1016/s0016-5085(99)70507-x. PMID: 10348826.

[57] Corica D, Romano C. Renal Involvement in Inflammatory Bowel Diseases. J Crohns Colitis. 2016 Feb;10(2):226-235. doi: 10.1093/ecco-jcc/jjv138. Epub 2015 Jul 29. PMID: 26223844.

[58] Gaspar SR, Mendonça T, Oliveira P, Oliveira T, Dias J, Lopes T. Urolithiasis and crohn's disease. Urol Ann. 2016 Jul-Sep;8(3):297-304. doi: 10.4103/0974-7796.184879. PMID: 27453651; PMCID: PMC4944622.

[59] Cirillo M, Iudici M, Marcarelli F, Laudato M, Zincone F. La nefrolitiasi nelle malattie intestinali [Nephrolithiasis in patients with intestinal diseases]. G Ital Nefrol. 2008 Jan-Feb;25(1):42–8. Italian. PMID: 18264917.

[60] Choi JY, Yu CH, Jung HY, Jung MK, Kim YJ, Cho JH, Kim CD, Kim YL, Park SH. A case of rapidly progressive IgA nephropathy in a patient with exacerbation of Crohn's disease. BMC Nephrol. 2012 Aug 6;13:84. doi: 10.1186/1471-2369-13-84. PMID: 22866754; PMCID: PMC3724487.

[61] Díaz Rodríguez C, Granja E, Vázquez Martul E, Sacristán F, Moreno Fernández A, González Rivero C, del Río Romero D, Trinidad JC. Asociación de glomerulonefritis membranosa y enfermedad de Crohn [Association between membranous glomerulonephritis and Crohn's disease]. Nefrologia. 2004;24(4):368-71. Spanish. PMID: 15455498.

[62] Izzedine H, Simon J, Piette AM, Lucsko M, Baumelou A, Charitanski D, Kernaonet E, Baglin AC, Deray G,

Beaufils H. Primary chronic interstitial nephritis in Crohn's disease. Gastroenterology. 2002 Nov;123(5): 1436-1440. doi: 10.1053/ gast.2002.36613. PMID: 12404216.

[63] Saitoh O, Kojima K, Teranishi T, Nakagawa K, Kayazawa M, Nanri M, Egashira Y, Hirata I, Katsu Ki KI. Renal amyloidosis as a late complication of Crohn's disease: a case report and review of the literature from Japan. World J Gastroenterol. 2000 Jun;6(3): 461-464. doi: 10.3748/wjg.v6.i3.461. PMID: 11819631; PMCID: PMC4688785.

[64] Aarestrup J, Jess T, Kobylecki CJ, Nordestgaard BG, Allin KH. Cardiovascular Risk Profile Among Patients With Inflammatory Bowel Disease: A Population-based Study of More Than 100 000 Individuals. J Crohns Colitis. 2019 Mar 26;13(3): 319-323. doi: 10.1093/ecco-jcc/jjy164. PMID: 30321330.

[65] Mitchell NE, Harrison N, Junga Z, Singla M. Heart Under Attack: Cardiac Manifestations of Inflammatory Bowel Disease. Inflamm Bowel Dis. 2018 Oct 12;24(11):2322-2326. doi: 10.1093/ibd/ izy157. PMID: 29788235.

[66] Merceron O, Bailly C, Khalil A, Pontnau F, Hammoudi N, Dorent R, Michel PL. Mesalamine-induced myocarditis. Cardiol Res Pract. 2010 Sep 13;2010:930190. doi: 10.4061/2010/ 930190. PMID: 20871830; PMCID: PMC2943131.

[67] Uchida W, Mutsuga M, Ito H, Oshima H, Usui A. Nonbacterial Thrombotic Endocarditis Associated With Crohn Disease. Ann Thorac Surg. 2018 May;105(5):e199-e201. doi: 10.1016/j.athoracsur.2017.12.005. Epub 2018 Jan 3. PMID: 29305852.

[68] Hatoum OA, Binion DG, Otterson MF, Gutterman DD. Acquired microvascular dysfunction in inflammatory bowel disease: Loss of nitric oxide-mediated vasodilation. Gastroenterology. 2003 Jul;125(1):58-69. doi: 10.1016/s0016-5085(03)00699-1. PMID: 12851871.

[69] Giannotta M, Tapete G, Emmi G, Silvestri E, Milla M. Thrombosis in inflammatory bowel diseases: what's the link? Thromb J. 2015 Apr 2;13:14. doi: 10.1186/s12959-015-0044-2. PMID: 25866483; PMCID: PMC4393581.

[70] Tagle M, Barriga J, Piñeiro A. Enfermedad de Crohn asociada a la lesion pulmonar focal [Crohn's disease associated with focal pulmonare lesion]. Rev Gastroenterol Peru. 2003 Oct-Dec; 23(4):293–6. Spanish. PMID: 14716424.

[71] Mikhaĭlova ZF, Levchenko SV, Karagodina IuIa, Barinov VV. [Pulmonary disorders in patients with chronic inflammatory bowel disease]. Eksp Klin Gastroenterol. 2011;(3):54-9. Russian. PMID: 21695953.

[72] Wallaert B, Colombel JF, Tonnel AB, Bonniere P, Cortot A, Paris JC, Voisin C. Evidence of lymphocyte alveolitis in Crohn's disease. Chest. 1985 Mar;87(3):363-367. doi: 10.1378/chest.87.3.363. PMID: 3971763.

[73] Mikhaĭlova ZF, Parfenov AI, Ruchkina IN, Rogozina VA. [External respiratory function in patients with Crohn's disease]. Eksp Klin Gastroenterol. 2011;(2):82-5. Russian. PMID: 21560645.

[74] Tzanakis N, Bouros D, Samiou M, Panagou P, Mouzas J, Manousos O, Siafakas N. Lung function in patients with inflammatory bowel disease. Respir Med. 1998 Mar;92(3):516-522. doi: 10.1016/s0954-6111(98)90301-8. PMID: 9692115.

[75] Iwama T, Higuchi T, Imajo M, Akagawa S, Matsubara O, Mishima Y. Tracheo-bronchitis as a complication of Crohn's disease–a case report. Jpn J Surg. 1991 Jul;21(4):454-457. doi: 10.1007/BF02470975. PMID: 1960905.

[76] Butland RJ, Cole P, Citron KM, Turner-Warwick M. Chronic bronchial suppuration and inflammatory bowel disease. Q J Med. 1981;50(197):63-75. PMID: 7267968.

[77] Gil-Simón P, Barrio Andrés J, Atienza Sánchez R, Julián Gómez L, López Represa C, Caro-Patón A. Bronquiolitis obliterante con neumonía organizada y enfermedad de Crohn [Bronchiolitis obliterans organizing pneumonia and Crohn's disease]. Rev Esp Enferm Dig. 2008 Mar;100(3):175–7. Spanish. doi: 10.4321/s1130-01082008000300010. PMID: 18416645.

[78] Golpe R, Mateos A, Pérez-Valcárcel J, Lapeña JA, García-Figueiras R, Blanco J. Multiple pulmonary nodules in a patient with Crohn's disease. Respiration. 2003 May-Jun;70(3): 306-309. doi: 10.1159/000072015. PMID: 12915753.

[79] Patwardhan RV, Heilpern RJ, Brewster AC, Darrah JJ. Pleuropericarditis: an extraintestinal complication of inflammatory bowel disease. Report of three cases and review of literature. Arch Intern Med. 1983 Jan;143(1):94-96. PMID: 6849612.

[80] Sostman HD, Matthay RA, Putman CE, Smith GJ. Methotrexate-induced pneumonitis. Medicine (Baltimore). 1976 Sep;55(5):371-388. doi: 10.1097/00005792-197609000-00002. PMID: 957997.

[81] Gupta A, Gulati S. Mesalamine induced eosinophilic pneumonia. Respir Med Case Rep. 2017 Apr 12;21:116-117. doi: 10.1016/j.rmcr.2017.04.010. PMID: 28458997; PMCID: PMC5397013.

[82] Keane J, Gershon S, Wise RP, Mirabile-Levens E, Kasznica J, Schwieterman WD, Siegel JN, Braun MM. Tuberculosis associated with infliximab, a tumor necrosis factor alpha-neutralizing agent. N Engl J Med. 2001 Oct 11;345(15):1098-1104. doi: 10.1056/NEJMoa011110. PMID: 11596589.

[83] Stratakos G, Kalomenidis I, Papas V, Malagari K, Kollintza A, Roussos C, Anagnostopoulou M, Paniara O, Zakynthinos S, Papiris SA. Cough and fever in a female with Crohn's disease receiving infliximab. Eur Respir J. 2005 Aug;26(2):354-357. doi: 10.1183/09031936.05.00005205. PMID: 16055885.

[84] Colombel JF, Loftus EV Jr, Tremaine WJ, Egan LJ, Harmsen WS, Schleck CD, Zinsmeister AR, Sandborn WJ. The safety profile of infliximab in patients with Crohn's disease: the Mayo clinic experience in 500 patients. Gastroenterology. 2004 Jan;126(1):19-31. doi: 10.1053/j.gastro.2003.10.047. PMID: 14699483.

Chapter 3

Recent Advances in Diagnosis and Management of Crohn's Disease

Anjana Bali and Monika Rani

Abstract

The initiation of Crohn's disease, an inflammatory bowel disease, has been primarily associated with crypt inflammation and abscesses, which further progresses towards the development of mucosal lesion and ulcers followed by mucosal edema. Despite many years of research for the confirmatory role of inflammation in this disease, various pathways and diagnosis for this inflammatory cascade is still unrevealed, which in fact is of utmost importance in the assessment of disease activity and for tailoring the therapy. Till now, various histopathological as well as endoscopic examinations has been found to be effectively and accurately assess inflammatory activity, but they are invasive, time consuming and expensive and therefore are unsuitable for routine use. Consequently, the latest research is focusing on various biomarkers of intestinal inflammation and the corresponding biological therapy. So, this chapter will cover the recent advances in diagnosis and pharmacological therapies for the same.

Keywords: inflammation, biological therapy, fibrostenosis, stricture, immune response

1. Introduction

Crohn's disease (CD) is a chronic, inflammatory disease, mainly affecting the gastro-intestinal tract and is usually characterized as relapse-remitting condition with progressive bowel damage [1, 2]. Being first discovered in 1932 in the United States, its rising prevalence in Europe, North America and developing countries of East Asia and South America during the 20th century is of serious health concern [3–6]. The complex etiology of CD is still unresolved and the pathogenesis is supposed to involve various genetic, environmental, gut-mucosal and immune-mediated factors which ultimately causing the initiation of inflammatory cascade followed by altered epithelial barrier function and mucosal damage [7–9]. CD represents bowel inflammation at the time of diagnosis but with disease progression, various complications such as fibrotic stenosis and strictures occur which lead to the bowel blockages [10]. Several cohort studies have reported that in about 80% of the patients, CD is characterized by inflammation and approximately 5–28% of them presents with fibrotic structuring [11–13]. Also, in case of CD complications, the additional surgery cost presents a huge socioeconomic burden in developed as well as developing countries [6, 14].

The diagnosis of crohn's disease (CD) in clinical settings is still challenging because of the lack of accuracy and specificity of the currently available diagnostic tools, various serological, genetic and inflammatory biomarkers. Also the heterogeneous nature of various fibrotic and inflammatory pathways involved in the disease limits the scope of such techniques [15, 16]. Preceding the inaccessibility towards the deep fibrotic site while using the invasive, expensive and time consuming conventional endoscopy, several advances have been made in the diagnosis of CD from both diagnostic and therapeutic perspectives. Diagnosis, disease activity, and therapeutic response are currently assessed by endoscopy, cross-sectional imaging, and biomarkers. Furthermore, because of paucity of effective drugs to treat inflammatory as well as complicated CD, a step-up approach of therapeutic management is required to not only to decrease disease activity but also to improve quality of life of the suffering population in clinical practice. Considering these points, this book chapter will discuss the recent advances in diagnosis and management of CD.

2. Diagnostic approach

2.1 Endoscopy and serological tests

Till now, the diagnostic process in clinical settings completely relied on various conventional techniques such as endoscopy and serological tests [7, 17]. Various antibodies against microbial antigens such as anti-Saccharomyces Cerevisiae antibodies (ASCA), outer membrane porin (anti-OmpC), flagellin (anti-Cbir1), and Pseudomonas flourescens- associated sequence 1–2 (anti-12) etcetera has been found to be involved in altered microbial biota in CD patients. IgA anti-OmpC, IgG anti-Cbir1 and IgA anti-I2 were found to be positive in approximately 55% of CD cases [18–20]. Furthermore, the elevated serum levels of various new antiglycan antibodies such as anti-aminaribioside (ALCA), anti-mannobioside carbohydrate antibody (AMCA) and anti-chitobioside carbohydrate antibody (ACCA) in CD patients has been remained an indicator for these antibodies as diagnostic biomarkers in patients suffering from CD [21]. A meta- analysis by Kaul et al., 2012, reported positive correlation between the number of positive anti-glycan antibodies and disease severity [22].

2.2 Inflammatory markers

As inflammation plays a prominent role in the initiation and progression of Crohn's disease, so determination of inflammatory state is crucial for the assessment of disease activity and for tailoring therapy. Non-invasive inflammatory markers such as C-reactive protein (CRP) and erythrocyte sedimentation rate (ESR) have been used for these indications. CRP, an acute phase protein, produced primarily by hepatocytes in response to inflammatory trigger mediated by various other cytokines such as interleukin-6 (IL-6) and tumor necrosis factor (TNF)-α, has proven its role as inflammatory biomarker from past decades but has since fallen out of favor as they are generally non-specific. More recently, markers of inflammation that are specific to the GI tract, such as fecal calprotectin (FC) and stool lactoferrin (SL), have been introduced as well established biomarker of intestinal inflammation. Various studies have reported the positive correlation between increased levels of FC and CD progression [23, 24]. In addition another research has documented that the increased levels of CRP, ESR in combination with fecal calprotectin proves best biomarker for the early diagnosis of crohn's disease in children suffering from abdominal pain and diarrhea [25]. Apart from this, various genetic biomarkers have evolved their role not only in the etiology of disease but also play a role in the disease pathogenesis as well as phenotype. Among genetic markers, the functional polymorphs of the interferon regulatory factor 5 (IRF5) were found to affect the risk profile for CD [26]. The assessment of serological biomarkers and inflammatory biomarkers as an adjunct to genetic biomarkers such as extracellular matrix protein −1 (ECM1), signal transducer and activator of transcription 3 (STAT3) etcetera could help in the early diagnosis of complications associated with [27].

2.3 Advanced imaging techniques

Imaging techniques provides the platform not only to understand the pathology of the disease but are also able to provide detailed note about the molecular mechanism involved in the disease, thus helps in aiding better therapeutic decisions about the disease. Among conventional techniques, Barium follow-through (BaFT) has been used to diagnose luminal small bowel CD [28]. Nowadays, these have been replaced by new endoscopic developments such as double balloon endoscopy and capsule endoscopy as BaFTs assess only the intraluminal mucosal pathology, meanwhile obscuring the lesion caused by superimposition of the bowel loops. The development of cross-sectional imaging technologies facilitates the accurate and rapid assessment of not only the small bowel and adjacent tissues but also assess deep layers for strictures and extraintestinal complications such as abscesses & fistulas. Also the shift from techniques causing exposure of ionizing radiation such as computerized tomography (CT), towards safe non-radiating, non-invasive, cost efficient and safe cross sectional techniques such as ultrasound (US) and magnetic resonance imaging (MRI) have changed the clinical perspective towards the disease complication. The modified version of these techniques such as computerized tomography enterography (CTE), intestinal ultrasound (IUS), magnetic resonance enterography (MRE), contrast enhanced ultrasonography (CEUS) etcetera has been preferred diagnostic tools even for the early prediction of CD complications [29, 30].

2.3.1 Computed tomography enterography (CTE)

After its discovery in 1977 to assess the extent and severity of CD, CTE has evolved its role in the diagnosis of intraluminal and extraintestinal complications involved in CD patients [31, 32]. Moreover, it differs from the conventional abdominal CT scan techniques in a way that it involves the intake of enteric or oral contrast medium to achieve adequate luminal distension [33]. This technique involves the use of small bowel distension along with the mixture of low density or neutral contrast agents and an abdominal CT examination following the administration of intravenous contrast agents [29]. Apart from enabling the dynamic imaging, CTE provides additional advantages such as lower cost, lesser influence of bowel peristalsis, wide availability, and greater patient safety with lesser need of general anesthesia and better efficacy in patients sensitive to MRI [31]. However, the use of ionizing radiation make its use little disadvantageous but various new techniques has been developed which makes CT examinations at significantly lesser radiation rate in pediatrics and adolescents [34–36].

2.3.2 Small bowel ultrasound (SBUS)

This inexpensive, non-radiating and well-tolerated technique provides detailed evaluation of bowel and abdominal viscera [37]. This technique has been preferred for pediatric and young non-obese patients as obesity obscure the thorough examination. Irrespective of its dependency for use on special training and practice, it is still considered comparable to endoscopy and MRE [38, 39].

2.3.3 Magnetic resonance enterography (MRE)

As per the American College of Radiology's Appropriateness Criteria, MRE has become first line of choice for evaluating children or young patients of CD [40]. Also a recent study has demonstrated its greater sensitivity and specificity as compared to US and its superiority for disease mapping over other techniques [41]. Several studies have compared the use of CTE and MRE and reported that both the techniques have similar sensitivities and specificities in diagnosing CD [29, 42]. MRE has been reported to be more advantageous because of absence of ionizing radiations, high tissue contrast resolution, and less adverse effects because of use of intravenous contrast materials [29]. However, MRE technique also has some disadvantages including longer acquisition time, hindrance due to peristalsis and bowel movements and it has been found to be more expensive, time-consuming, and less well-tolerated than SBUS and CTE [31, 43].

Thus proteomics has emerged as an attractive approach not only to define the pathogenesis of disease but also to distinguish inflammatory and fibrostenotic phenotypes and predict the complications at an earliest. Coupling these protein biomarkers through proteomics with various non-invasive, non-radiating imaging techniques may aid in better diagnosis of CD and may provide a novel approach for the treatment of CD.

3. Therapy approach

3.1 Conventional therapeutic approach

The etiology and pathogenesis of CD is still complex and unresolved, curbing the development of new therapeutic agents for its treatment. The remission and recurrence of disease demands the effective induction and maintenance therapy while reducing the disease complications and improving the quality of life. Till date, aminosalicyclic acids, corticosteroids and various immunomodulators has been considered as therapeutic agents of choice, but lack of efficacy because of heterogenecity of disease and higher toxicity profile of these drugs have made these drugs inappropriate.

Among aminosalicylates, sulfasalazine and mesalamine has been effective in the treatment of CD. Various clinical studies have reported the role of sulfasalazine (3–6 gm/day) in the remission of mild to moderate CD [44, 45]. Mesalamine has been used routinely for decades in patients with Crohn's disease in clinical practice. A recent study have demonstrated that mesalamine at doses above 2.4 g/d was more effective than placebo for the induction of remission of Crohn's disease [46], but owing to less benefits, this class has gone out of favor in clinical practice [47]. Even various systematic reviews and meta-analyses remained inconclusive about the role of ASA in remission of active CD and preventing relapse of CD [48, 49]. Furthermore, broad spectrum antibiotics have been considered to be clinically efficacious as compared to narrow spectrum since the strain of intestinal bacteria involved in the progression of CD is still uncertain [50]. So, various clinical trials have reported the efficacy of antibiotics such as metronidazole, ciprofloxacin, clarithrmycin, rifaximin and anti-tuberculous regimen for the treatment of mild to moderately active CD [51, 52]. Rifaximin have shown its efficacy against majority of intestinal flora with relatively infrequent bacterial resistance. On the same pace, it has shown its effectiveness in CD with ciprofloxacin 500 mg, orally twice daily, given for the duration of 6 months [53]. Furthermore, a randomized controlled trial has shown the significant clinical efficacy with metronidazole [54]. As per recent study, low-dose metronidazole in dose of 250 mg t.i.d. for the duration of 3 months even reduces the endoscopic postoperative recurrence rates in crohn's disease [55]. Moreover, Metronidazole in combination with ciprofloxacin 500 mg bid have shown promising rate of remission [56]. Furthermore, rifaximin, another broad spectrum antibiotic was found to be efficacious in various clinical trials. The double blind randomized controlled trials (RCT) were conducted by Prantera and coworkers 2006 & 2010. In these RCT's, 83 patients having 800 b.i.d. dose & 402 patients having 400–1200 b.i.d dose respectively for the duration of 3 months, have shown promising remission rate in CD [57, 58]. Various other studies have also demonstrated the same effects of rifaximin, in the dose of 800 mg b.i.d for the duration of 3 months [52, 59, 60].

Furthermore, corticosteroids were included in the algorithm of CD therapy. An accumulative body of literature has reported the preference of corticosteroid efficacy over conventional steroids and ASA's in CD, especially for ileocecal and ileal diseases [61–63]. Budesonide in combination with ciprofloxacin and metronidazole have shown effectiveness in induction of remission in CD patients but again the higher frequency of serious adverse reactions do not favor their use as routine therapy [64]. Moreover, the available data are limited to small uncontrolled trials that have not consistently demonstrated efficacy with these agents at inducing clinical remission for mild to moderate CD [54]. In addition, they are associated with a high potential for dependence and serious adverse effects [62, 65]. So, the rising detrimental effects of corticosteroids, which once has been used as first line therapy from the past decades, has led to stringent attempts to limit their use in the treatment of CD.

3.2 Advanced therapeutic approach

CD pathogenesis involves the breaching of epithelial barrier of mucosal layer and luminal microflora tend to stimulate the pro-inflammatory immune response leading to release of various proinflammatory cytokines such as interferon-gamma, interleukin 12, TNF- α and [66, 67]. Biologics therapy has been approved by FDA for the treatment of inflammatory cascade long time ago but the discovery of new molecules in this arena is still continued and represents a major breakthrough in the treatment of CD. The advanced therapeutic approach includes biologic agents such as immunomodulators, anti-TNF- α agents, IL-12, IL-23 antagonists, anti-adhesion molecules and monoclonal antibodies. Immunomodulators has been used primarily for inflammatory state of CD in clinical practice from many years. Among immunomodulators, Azathioprine (AZA) and 6-mercaptopurine (6-MP) has been included in the meta-analysis studies and have revealed their role in the remission in CD patients but with occurrence of serious adverse effects [68, 69]. On the other side, biologicals such as TNF-α antagonists and IL antagonists have been adopted for the treatment of CD complications such as fistulas and strictures. Moreover, these offer advantage over corticosteroids which tend to suppress the entire immune system and produce various adverse effects. Biologics target the inflammatory pathway specifically, with lesser unpredictable side effects. The US Food & Drug Administration (FDA) approved infliximab in 1998, followed by the approval of adalimumab and certolizumab. These TNF-α antagonist remained as an effective option among biologics since now for the treatment of CD. Systematic reviews and meta-analyses have evidenced about the role of adalimumab and infliximab in the maintenance and remission of CD [70–72]. Moreover, various optimization strategies have been given regarding the use of anti-TNF agents in CD patients. Likewise, as per SONIC study, infliximab was found to be more efficacious when given in combination with azathioprine as compared to monotherapy [73]. Although

TNF-antagonist therapy has greatly improved the management of CD, these drugs have some important limitations [74, 75]. Also, Up to one-third of patients do not respond to induction therapy, and an additional 40% lose response over the first year [76]. Treatment with a second TNF antagonist in patients failing these agents has only modest efficacy [77]. Thus, a need exists for alternative therapies. So, in recent years, a range of newer molecules has been discovered and implemented in clinical practice. Among these agents, Vedolizumab and Ustekinumab have shown effective and safe profile in the induction and remission of CD [78, 79]. Vedolizumab, the selective leukocyte adhesion molecule inhibitor was approved for CD in 2014, followed by ustekinumab, the monoclonal antibody that targets interleukin-12 and interleukin-23 in 2016. Furthermore, Pirfenidone and nintedanib which have been used for the treatment of pulmonary fibrosis have also proven their role in the management of fibrostenotic CD [80, 81]. Considering the efficacy of combination of immunomodulators with biologicals, it has been reported that inflixmab prescribed along with thiopurines is more efficacious as compared to infliximab alone or thiopurines alone [82].

Thus, 5-Aminosalicylic acid agents are not considered as first choice for treatment of CD. Corticosteroids such as Budesonide and Prednisone are now-a-days considered as the first line agents. Broad spectrum antibiotics such as metronidazole, ciprofloxacin, clarithrmycin and rifaximin have been considered to be clinically efficacious and remained as important adjuncts for the treatment of mild CD. Immunomodulators are used as second line agents in mild to moderate Crohn's disease. They act by modifying the immune system while inducing and maintaining remission. Biologicals such as Adalimumab, Infliximab, certolizumab, Vedolizumab eand Ustekinumab are used in moderate to severely active CD.

4. Conclusions

On concluding remarks, the diagnosis as well as management of CD and associated complications should remain the ultimate goal. From diagnostic perspective, CTE and MRE are at the forefront and providing new ways to quantify disease activity in order to provide more personalized therapy in clinical practice. Furthermore, from the diagnostic perspectives, the continuous evolvement of biologicals such as anti TNF-α and IL-antagonists has been proven as revolution in the treatment of inflammation as well as various complications associated with CD. Although the current therapy available for CD meets the safety as well as efficacy data requirements, still there is need of newer agents with high efficacy, less side effects and improved pharmacodynamic as well as pharmacokinetic profile. So, the anticipated discovery of new diagnostic biomarkers and therapeutic agents while minimizing the use of conventional endoscopic and radiologic examination will enable physicians to provide individualized treatment plans in order to improve the long-term prognosis of patients suffering from CD.

Conflict of interest

The authors declare no conflict of interest.

Author details

Anjana Bali[1] and Monika Rani[2]*

1 Central University of Punjab, Bathinda, Punjab, India

2 Chitkara University, Patiala, Punjab, India

*Address all correspondence to: monika.rani@chitkara.edu.in

References

[1] Freeman HJ. Natural history and long-term clinical course of Crohn's disease. World journal of gastroenterology: WJG. 2014;20(1):31.

[2] Baumgart DC, Sandborn WJ. Crohn's disease. Lancet 2012;380:1590e605

[3] Kotze PG, Underwood FE, Damião AO, Ferraz JG, Saad-Hossne R, Toro M, Iade B, Bosques-Padilla F, Teixeira FV, Juliao-Banos F, Simian D. Progression of inflammatory bowel diseases throughout Latin America and the Caribbean: a systematic review. Clinical Gastroenterology and Hepatology. 2020;18(2):304-312.

[4] Kaplan GG. The global burden of IBD: from 2015 to 2025. Nature reviews Gastroenterology & hepatology. 2015;12(12):720-727.

[5] Prideaux L, Kamm MA, De Cruz PP, Chan FK, Ng SC. Inflammatory bowel disease in Asia: a systematic review. Journal of gastroenterology and hepatology. 2012;27(8):1266-1280.

[6] Goh KL, XIAO SD. Inflammatory bowel disease: a survey of the epidemiology in Asia. Journal of digestive diseases. 2009 ;10(1):1-6.

[7] Gajendran M, Loganathan P, Catinella AP, Hashash JG. A comprehensive review and update on Crohn's disease. Disease-a-month. 2018;64(2):20-57.

[8] De Souza HS, Fiocchi C. Immunopathogenesis of IBD: current state of the art. Nature reviews Gastroenterology & hepatology. 2016;13(1):13.

[9] Liu JZ, Anderson CA. Genetic studies of Crohn's disease: past, present and future. Best Practice & Research Clinical Gastroenterology. 2014;28(3):373-386.

[10] Chan WP, Mourad F, Leong RW. Crohn's disease associated strictures. Journal of gastroenterology and hepatology. 2018;33(5):998-1008.

[11] Rieder F, Zimmermann EM, Remzi FH, Sandborn WJ. Crohn's disease complicated by strictures: a systematic review. Gut. 2013;62: 1072-1084.

[12] Henriksen M, Jahnsen J, Lygren I, Aadland E, Schulz T, Vatn MH, Moum B, Ibsen Study Group. Clinical course in Crohn's disease: results of a five-year population-based follow-up study (the IBSEN study). Scandinavian journal of gastroenterology. 2007;42(5):602-610.

[13] Papi C, Festa V, Fagnani C, Stazi A, Antonelli G, Moretti A, Koch M, Capurso L. Evolution of clinical behaviour in Crohn's disease: predictive factors of penetrating complications. Digestive and liver disease. 2005;37(4):247-253.

[14] Bodger K, Kikuchi T, Hughes D. Cost-effectiveness of biological therapy for Crohn's disease: Markov cohort analyses incorporating United Kingdom patient-level cost data. Alimentary pharmacology & therapeutics. 2009;30(3):265-274.

[15] Cappello M, Morreale GC. The role of laboratory tests in Crohn's disease. Clinical Medicine Insights: Gastroenterology. 2016:CGast-S38203.

[16] Woo MH, Cho YH, Sohn MJ, Lee EJ, Kim JW, Moon JS, Ko JS, Kim HY. Use of Anti-TNF Alpha Blockers Can Reduce Operation Rate and Lead to Growth Gain in Pediatric Crohn's Disease. Pediatric gastroenterology, hepatology & nutrition. 2019;22(4):358-368.

[17] Gomollon F, Dignass A, Annese V, Tilg H, Van Assche G, Lindsay JO,

Peyrin-Biroulet L, Cullen GJ, Daperno M, Kucharzik T, Rieder F. 3rd European evidence-based consensus on the diagnosis and management of Crohn's disease 2016: part 1: diagnosis and medical management. Journal of Crohn's and Colitis. 2017;11(1):3-25.

[18] Mokrowiecka A, Daniel P, Slomka M, Majak P, Malecka-Panas E. Clinical utility of serological markers in inflammatory bowel disease. Hepatogastroenterology. 2009;56:162-166.

[19] Lodes MJ, Cong Y, Elson CO, Mohamath R, Landers CJ, Targan SR, Fort M, Hershberg RM. Bacterial flagellin is a dominant antigen in Crohn disease. The Journal of clinical investigation. 2004;113(9):1296-1306.

[20] Landers CJ, Cohavy O, Misra R, Yang H, Lin YC, Braun J, Targan SR. Selected loss of tolerance evidenced by Crohn' s disease-associated immune responses to auto- and microbial antigens. Gastroenterology 2002; 123: 689-699.

[21] Iborra M, Beltran B, Nos P. Noninvasive testing for mucosal inflammation in inflammatory bowel disease. Gastrointestinal Endoscopy Clinics. 2016;26(4):641-656.

[22] Kaul A, Hutfless S, Liu L, Bayless TM, Marohn MR, Li X. Serum anti-glycan antibody biomarkers for inflammatory bowel disease diagnosis and progression: a systematic review and meta-analysis. Inflammatory bowel diseases. 2012;18(10):1872-1884.

[23] Kennedy NA, Jones GR, Plevris N, Patenden R, Arnott ID, Lees CW. Association between level of fecal calprotectin and progression of Crohn's disease. Clinical Gastroenterology and Hepatology. 2019;17(11):2269-2276.

[24] Bjarnason I. The use of fecal calprotectin in inflammatory bowel disease. Gastroenterology & hepatology. 2017;13(1):53.

[25] Daniluk U, Daniluk J, Krasnodebska M, Lotowska JM, Sobaniec-Lotowska ME, Lebensztejn DM. The combination of fecal calprotectin with ESR, CRP and albumin discriminates more accurately children with Crohn's disease. Advances in medical sciences. 2019;64(1):9-14.

[26] Gathungu G, Zhang CK, Zhang W, Cho JH. A two-marker haplotype in the IRF5 gene is associated with inflammatory bowel disease in a North American cohort. Genes & Immunity. 2012;13(4):351-355.

[27] Lichtenstein GR, Targan SR, Dubinsky MC, Rotter JI, Barken DM, Princen F, Carroll S, Brown M, Stachelski J, Chuang E, Landers CJ. Combination of genetic and quantitative serological immune markers are associated with complicated Crohn's disease behavior. Inflammatory bowel diseases. 2011;17(12):2488-2496.

[28] Hafeez R, Greenhalgh R, Rajan J, Bloom S, McCartney S, Halligan S, Taylor SA. Use of small bowel imaging for the diagnosis and staging of Crohn's disease-a survey of current UK practice. The British Journal of Radiology. 2011;84(1002):508-517.

[29] Kim SH. Computed tomography enterography and magnetic resonance enterography in the diagnosis of Crohn's disease. Intestinal Research. 2015;13(1):27.

[30] Bourreille A, Ignjatovic A, Aabakken L, Loftus Jr EV, Eliakim R, Pennazio M, Bouhnik Y, Seidman E, Keuchel M, Albert JG, Ardizzone S. Role of small-bowel endoscopy in the management of patients with inflammatory bowel disease: an international OMED-ECCO consensus. 2009:618-637.

[31] Hammer MR, Podberesky DJ, Dillman JR. Multidetector computed tomographic and magnetic resonance enterography in children: state of the art. Radiologic Clinics. 2013;51(4):615-636.

[32] Ilangovan R, Burling D, George A, Gupta A, Marshall M, Taylor SA. CT enterography: review of technique and practical tips. The British journal of radiology. 2012;85(1015):876-886.

[33] Paulsen SR, Huprich JE, Fletcher JG, Booya F, Young BM, Fidler JL, Johnson CD, Barlow JM, Earnest IV F. CT enterography as a diagnostic tool in evaluating small bowel disorders: review of clinical experience with over 700 cases. Radiographics. 2006;26(3):641-657.

[34] Craig O, O'Neill S, O'Neill F, McLaughlin P, McGarrigle A, McWilliams S, O'Connor O, Desmond A, Walsh EK, Ryan M, Maher M. Diagnostic accuracy of computed tomography using lower doses of radiation for patients with Crohn's disease. Clinical gastroenterology and hepatology. 2012;10(8):886-892.

[35] Lee SJ, Park SH, Kim AY, Yang SK, Yun SC, Lee SS, Jung GS, Ha HK. A prospective comparison of standard-dose CT enterography and 50% reduced-dose CT enterography with and without noise reduction for evaluating Crohn disease. American Journal of Roentgenology. 2011;197(1):50-57.

[36] Kambadakone AR, Prakash P, Hahn PF, Sahani DV. Low-dose CT examinations in Crohn's disease: impact on image quality, diagnostic performance, and radiation dose. American journal of roentgenology. 2010;195(1):78-88.

[37] Panes J, Bouhnik Y, Reinisch W, Stoker J, Taylor SA, Baumgart DC, Danese S, Halligan S, Marincek B, Matos C, Peyrin-Biroulet L. Imaging techniques for assessment of inflammatory bowel disease: joint ECCO and ESGAR evidence-based consensus guidelines. Journal of Crohn's and Colitis. 2013;7(7):556-585.

[38] Jairath V, Ordas I, Zou G, Panes J, Stoker J, Taylor SA, Santillan C, Horsthuis K, Samaan MA, Shackelton LM, Stitt LW. Reliability of measuring ileo-colonic disease activity in crohn's disease by magnetic resonance enterography. Inflammatory bowel diseases. 2018;24(2):440-449.

[39] Marteau P, Laharie D, Colombel JF, Martin L, Coevoet H, Allez M, Cadiot G, Bourreille A, Carbonnel F, Bouhnik Y, Coffin B. Interobserver variation study of the Rutgeerts score to assess endoscopic recurrence after surgery for Crohn's disease. Journal of Crohn's and Colitis. 2016;10(9):1001-1005.

[40] Expert Panel on Gastrointestinal Imaging. American College of Radiology ACR Appropriateness Criteria: Crohn disease. 2011:1-17. Available from: http://www.acr.org/~/media/ACR/Documents/AppCriteria/Diagnostic/CrohnDisease.pdf.

[41] Taylor SA, Mallett S, Bhatnagar G, Baldwin-Cleland R, Bloom S, Gupta A, Hamlin PJ, Hart AL, Higginson A, Jacobs I, McCartney S. Diagnostic accuracy of magnetic resonance enterography and small bowel ultrasound for the extent and activity of newly diagnosed and relapsed Crohn's disease (METRIC): a multicentre trial. The lancet Gastroenterology & hepatology. 2018;3(8):548-558.

[42] Deepak P, Fletcher JG, Fidler JL, Bruining DH. Computed tomography and magnetic resonance enterography in Crohn's disease: assessment of radiologic criteria and endpoints for clinical practice and trials. Inflammatory bowel diseases. 2016;22(9):2280-2288.

[43] Miles A, Bhatnagar G, Halligan S, Gupta A, Tolan D, Zealley I, Taylor SA. Magnetic resonance enterography, small bowel ultrasound and colonoscopy to diagnose and stage Crohn's disease: patient acceptability and perceived burden. European radiology. 2019;29(3):1083-1093.

[44] Malchow H, Ewe K, Brandes JW, et al. European Cooperative Crohn's Disease Study (ECCDS): results of drug treatment. J Gastroenterol 1984;86:249-266.

[45] Van Hees PA, Van Lier HJ, Van Elteren PH, et al. Effect of sulphasalazine in patients with active Crohn's disease: a controlled double-blind study. Gut 1981;22:404-409.

[46] Coward S, Kuenzig ME, Hazlewood G, Clement F, McBrien K, Holmes R, Panaccione R, Ghosh S, Seow CH, Rezaie A, Kaplan GG. Comparative effectiveness of mesalamine, sulfasalazine, corticosteroids, and budesonide for the induction of remission in Crohn's disease: a Bayesian network meta-analysis. Inflammatory bowel diseases. 2017;23(3):461-472.

[47] Moja L, Danese S, Fiorino G, et al. Systematic review with network metaanalysis: comparative efficacy and safety of budesonide and mesalazine (mesalamine) for Crohn's disease. Aliment Pharmacol Ther. 2015;41:1055-1065.

[48] Ilheozor-Ejiofor Z, Gordon M, Clegg A, Freeman SC, Gjuladin-Hellon T, MacDonald JK, Akobeng AK. Interventions for maintenance of surgically induced remission in Crohn's disease: a network meta-analysis. Cochrane Database of Systematic Reviews. 2019;9.

[49] Ford AC, Kane SV, Khan KJ, Achkar JP, Talley NJ, Marshall JK, Moayyedi P. Efficacy of 5-aminosalicylates in Crohn's disease: systematic review and meta-analysis. American Journal of Gastroenterology. 2011;106(4):617-629.

[50] Prantera C, Scribano ML. Antibiotics and probiotics in inflammatory bowel disease: why, when, and how. Curr Opin Gastroenterol. 2009;25:329-333.

[51] Collyer R, Clancy A, Agrawal G, Borody TJ. Crohn's strictures open with anti-mycobacterial antibiotic therapy: A retrospective review. World Journal of Gastrointestinal Endoscopy. 2020;12(12):542.

[52] Jigaranu AO, Nedelciuc O, Blaj A, Badea M, Mihai C, Diculescu M, Cijevschi-Prelipcean C. Is rifaximin effective in maintaining remission in Crohn's disease? Dig Dis. 2014;32:378-383.

[53] Arnold GL, Beaves MR, Pryjdun VO, Mook WJ. Preliminary study of ciprofloxacin in active Crohn's disease. Inflamm Bowel Dis. 2002; 8:10-15.

[54] Sutherland L, Singleton J, Sessions J, Hanauer S, Krawitt E, Rankin G, Summers R, Mekhjian H, Greenberger N, Kelly M. Double blind, placebo controlled trial of metronidazole in Crohn's disease. Gut 1991; 32: 1071-1075.

[55] Glick LR, Sossenheimer PH, Ollech JE, Cohen RD, Hyman NH, Hurst RD, Rubin DT. Low-dose metronidazole is associated with a decreased rate of endoscopic recurrence of Crohn's disease after ileal resection: a retrospective cohort study. Journal of Crohn's and Colitis. 2019;13(9):1158-1162.

[56] Prantera C, Zannoni F, Scribano ML, et al. An antibiotic regimen for the treatment of active Crohn's disease: A randomized, controlled clinical trial of metronidazole

plus ciprofloxacin. Am J Gastroenterol. 1996;91:328-332.

[57] Prantera C, Lochs H, Campieri M, Scribano ML, Sturniolo GC, Castiglione F, Cottone M. Antibiotic treatment of Crohn' s disease: results of a multicentre, double blind, randomized, placebo-controlled trial with rifaximin. Aliment Pharmacol. Ther 2006; 23: 1117-1125.

[58] Prantera C, Lochs H, Giochetti P. Rifaximin-EIR (extended intestinal release) 400 mg tablets in the treatment of moderately active Crohn's disease: results of the international multicentre, randomised, double-blind, placebo-controlled trial RETIC-03. Gut. 2010;59(Suppl III):A1.

[59] Prantera C, Lochs H, Grimaldi M, Danese S, Scribano ML, Gionchetti P. Rifaximin-extended intestinal release induces remission in patients with moderately active Crohn's disease. Gastroenterology 2012; 142: 473-481.e4.

[60] Khan KJ, Ullman TA, Ford AC, Abreu MT, Abadir A, Marshall JK, Nitzan O et al. Antibiotic therapy in inflammatory bowel disease: a systematic review and meta-analysis. Am J Gastroenterol 2011; 106: 661-673.

[61] Yokoyama T, Ohta A, Motoya S, Takazoe M, Yajima T, Date M, Nii M, Nagy P, Suzuki Y, Hibi T. Efficacy and safety of oral budesonide in patients with active crohn's disease in Japan: A multicenter, double-blind, randomized, parallel-group phase 3 study. Inflammatory intestinal diseases. 2017;2(3):154-162.

[62] Rezaie A, Kuenzig ME, Benchimol EI, Griffiths AM, Otley AR, Steinhart AH, Kaplan GG, Seow CH. Budesonide for induction of remission in Crohn's disease. Cochrane Database of Systematic Reviews. 2015(6).

[63] Greenberg GR, Feagan BG, Martin F, et al. Oral budesonide for active Crohn's disease. Canadian Inflammatory Bowel Disease Study Group. N Engl J Med 1994; 331:836-841.

[64] Steinhart AH, Feagan BG, Wong CJ, Vandervoort M, Mikolainis S, Croitoru K, Seidman E, Leddin DJ, Bitton A, Drouin E, Cohen A, Greenberg GR. Combined budesonide and antibiotic therapy for active Crohn's disease: a randomized controlled trial. Gastroenterology 2002; 123: 33-40.

[65] Kane SV, Schoenfeld P, Sandborn WJ, Tremaine W, Hofer T, Feagan BG. The effectiveness of budesonide therapy for Crohn's disease. 2002;16(8):1509-1517.

[66] Torres J., Mehandru S., Colombel JF., Peyrin-Biroulet L. Crohn's disease. Lancet 2017; 389:1741-1755.

[67] Sartor, R.B. Mechanisms of Disease: Pathogenesis of Crohn's disease and ulcerative colitis. Nat. Clin. Pract. Gastroenterol. Hepatol. 2006;3:390-407.

[68] Chande N, Tsoulis DJ, MacDonald JK. Azathioprine or 6-mercaptopurine for induction of remission in Crohn's disease. Cochrane database of systematic reviews. 2013(4).

[69] Pearson DC, May GR, Fick GH, Sutherland LR. Azathioprine and 6-mercaptopurine in Crohn disease: a meta-analysis. Annals of internal medicine. 1995;123(2):132-142.

[70] Dretzke J, Edlin R, Round J, Connock M, Hulme C, Czeczot J, Fry-Smith A, McCabe C, Meads C. A systematic review and economic evaluation of the use of tumour necrosis factor-alpha (TNF-α) inhibitors, adalimumab and infliximab, for Crohn's disease. Health Technology Assessment. 2011;15(6):1.

[71] Behm BW, Bickston SJ. Tumor necrosis factor-alpha antibody for maintenance of remission in Crohn's

disease. Cochrane Database of Systematic Reviews. 2008(1).

[72] Cassinotti A, Ardizzone S, Porro GB. Adalimumab for the treatment of Crohn's disease. Biologics: targets & therapy. 2008;2(4):763.

[73] Colombel JF, Sandborn WJ, Reinisch W, et al.; SONIC Study Group. Infliximab, azathioprine, or combination therapy for Crohn's disease. N Engl J Med. 2010;362:1383-1395.

[74] Singh JA, Wells GA, Christensen R, et al. Adverse effects of biologics: a network meta-analysis and Cochrane overview. Cochrane Database Syst Rev 2011:CD008794.

[75] Colombel JF, Sandborn WJ, Rutgeerts P, et al. Adalimumab for maintenance of clinical response and remission in patients with Crohn's disease: the CHARM trial. Gastroenterology 2007;132:52-65.

[76] Danese S, Fiorino G, Reinisch W. causative factors and the clinical management of patients with Crohn's disease who lose response to anti-TNF-α therapy. Alimentary pharmacology & therapeutics. 2011;34(1):10.

[77] Sandborn WJ, Rutgeerts P, Enns R, Hanauer SB, Colombel JF, Panaccione R, D'Haens G, Li J, Rosenfeld MR, Kent JD, Pollack PF. Adalimumab induction therapy for Crohn disease previously treated with infliximab: a randomized trial. Annals of internal medicine. 2007;146(12):829-838.

[78] Feagan BG, Sandborn WJ, Gasink C, Jacobstein D, Lang Y, Friedman JR, Blank MA, Johanns J, Gao LL, Miao Y, Adedokun OJ. Ustekinumab as induction and maintenance therapy for Crohn's disease. New England Journal of Medicine. 2016;375(20):1946-1960.

[79] Sandborn WJ, Feagan BG, Rutgeerts P, Hanauer S, Colombel JF, Sands BE, Lukas M, Fedorak RN, Lee S, Bressler B, Fox I. Vedolizumab as induction and maintenance therapy for Crohn's disease. New England Journal of Medicine. 2013;369(8):711-721.

[80] Rieder F, Fiocchi C, Rogler G. Mechanisms, management, and treatment of fibrosis in patients with inflammatory bowel diseases. Gastroenterology. 2017;152(2):340-350.

[81] Kadir SI, Wenzel Kragstrup T, Dige A, Kok Jensen S, Dahlerup JF, Kelsen J. Pirfenidone inhibits the proliferation of fibroblasts from patients with active Crohn's disease. Scandinavian journal of gastroenterology. 2016;51(11):1321-1325.

[82] Colombel JF, Sandborn WJ, Reinisch W, Mantzaris GJ, Kornbluth A, Rachmilewitz D, Lichtiger S, d'Haens G, Diamond RH, Broussard DL, Tang KL. Infliximab, azathioprine, or combination therapy for Crohn's disease. New England Journal of Medicine. 2010;362(15):1383-1395.

Chapter 4

Partial Enteral Nutrition in Crohn's Disease

Evgen Benedik, Darja Urlep, Anija Orel and Rok Orel

Abstract

Exclusive enteral nutrition (EEN) has proven to be a highly effective treatment option in inducing remission in active Crohn's disease (CD) in the paediatric population. In adults with CD, the results of meta-analyses demonstrated that therapy with corticosteroids was more effective in comparison with EEN. The most important limitation of the success of EEN treatment is patients' compliance. Exclusivity of enteral nutrition and its substantial impact on the quality of life are the main reasons why EEN is not acceptable to many patients. Therefore, the treatment with partial enteral nutrition (PEN), where patients are allowed to eat some ordinary food besides enteral formulas, is becoming an important treatment option, not only in inducing, but also in maintaining remission in CD. However, strong evidence on the efficacy of PEN for induction and maintenance of CD remission is still lacking. Due to the excellent safety profile of the treatment with enteral nutrition in comparison with other treatment modalities, further well-designed, randomised, controlled studies are necessary to elucidate the exact role of PEN in inducing and maintaining of remission in CD patients. Herein, the most relevant studies on the efficacy and the role of PEN in active and quiescent CD are reviewed.

Keywords: Crohn's disease, enteral nutrition, partial enteral nutrition, children, adults

1. Introduction

Crohn's disease (CD) is a life-long immune-mediated inflammatory disease which may affect any part of the gastrointestinal tract. The aetiology of the disease is multifactorial and complex, with genetic and environmental factors involved. It is widely accepted that inappropriate response of the innate and adaptive immune system to the altered composition of the indigenous intestinal microbiota plays crucial role in the pathogenesis. Both the development and treatment of the disease may therefore be influenced by different factors that can affect the composition of the intestinal microbiota, the permeability of the epithelial barrier, or the functioning of the gut immune system. Each of these factors can be significantly affected by nutrition. Epidemiological studies have shown that a diet containing large quantities of red and processed meat, animal fat, and refined sugars is associated with an increased risk, and a diet containing large quantities of fruits and vegetables with a reduced risk for CD development [1–4].

Therefore, the possibilities of treating CD with nutritional therapy are particularly interesting. Close partnership between the patients, gastroenterologist and dietitian is necessary when utilising nutritional therapy to treat CD. Dietitian provides support for dietary changes and asses the actual nutrient intake, patient's nutritional status, and discuss the role of enteral nutrition as the treatment option. Dietitian should be included in patient's treatment from diagnosis onwards. The ultimate goal of CD treatment is to induce and maintain clinical remission and mucosal healing with treatment modalities with least adverse effects [5]. Compared to other treatments such as corticosteroids (CS), immunomodulators and biologic drugs, nutritional therapy has an excellent safety profile, presenting with significantly less adverse effects compared to any other type of treatment. Many adverse effects of immunosuppressive drugs (thiopurines, methotrexate) and biological drugs, especially the increased risk of infections and malignancy, have been reported and are of major concern [6–9].

Since the discovery that exclusive enteral nutrition (EEN) that provides adequate nutritional intake of all macro- and micronutrients over a sufficiently long period can not only improve the nutritional status of patients but also alleviate inflammation, such treatment has been extensively studied. There is strong evidence that EEN is as effective as CS in inducing remission in patients with CD. In paediatric patients, when it comes to the induction of mucosal healing, EEN seems to be even more effective then CS [10–15]. EEN was also found to be able to promote transmural healing [16, 17]. There are currently many different enteral formulas available on the market. Some are elemental, semi-elemental and others polymeric. They differ in flavour, energy density, osmolarity, content of dietary fibre and some other nutrients but they all provide sufficient energy and essential nutrients intake.

Patients with CD are often malnourished at the time of diagnosis and growth retardation is frequently present in paediatric patients [18–20], so a positive effect on nutritional status and growth represents an important additional benefit of EEN [21]. Therefore, consensus guidelines of the European Society of Paediatric Gastroenterology, Hepatology and Nutrition (ESPGHAN) and the European Crohn's Colitis Organisation (ECCO) recommends EEN as a first-line therapy in all children with active CD, including those with colonic involvement [22]. Although, based on some initial studies, EEN had been shown to be as effective as CS for induction of remission also in adult patients with CD [23–27], subsequent studies did not confirmed this, and their meta-analyses demonstrated that CS were more effective treatment option in adult CD patients [13, 14, 28–31].

The reason for different efficacy of EEN in paediatric and adult CD populations is not completely understood. It may be due to longer disease course, higher prevalence of more aggressive phenotypes and more permanent structural changes of the bowel in adults. In addition, EEN is probably not so strictly adhered to in adult patients, when compared to children, who are usually under supervision from their parents. Children and especially adolescents are more motivated to achieve remission through the use of EEN, as most of them decline CS treatment due to appearance related side effects such as facies lunata, acne vulgaris and increased hairiness [5, 22]. The difference may also be due to the lack of well-designed randomised controlled studies in adult CD population. It has been noted, that the conclusions of the meta-analyses on the superior efficacy of CS in adults were mainly based on an intention to treat analyses, while when only results of the patients who strictly adhered to EEN protocols were analysed, the remission rates were comparable to those receiving CS [32]. Anyway, except for Japan, induction therapy with EEN is not common in adult patients with active CD. Japanese guidelines recommend EEN as one of the treatment options for active CD in adults [33], since a Japanese study reported that elemental EEN had a higher rate of induction of remission in CD patients compared with CS and has improved luminal lesions [34]. ECCO guidelines for medical management of adult CD from 2016 recommended the use of EEN as an adjunctive treatment to improve nutritional status and in patients who decline other drug therapy [35], while in the most recent edition of this guidelines from 2019 EEN is not mentioned at all [36]. Recent guidelines of the European Society for Clinical Nutrition and Metabolism (ESPEN) directly recommends EEN as a first line of treatment only for children and adolescents, while an option to use EEN in selected cases of adults is mentioned only in fine print [37].

Despite the strong evidence of EEN efficiency in paediatric and potentially in adult CD patients as well and its better impact on mucosal healing in comparison with CS, EEN is not popular in many parts of the world. Its major disadvantage is the need to consume exclusively enteral formulas, while avoiding all other foods for a long period, usually 6–8 weeks. This has a substantial impact on the quality of life and is unacceptable for many patients. Although all formulas used for EEN are designed for oral use, many patients (although there are significant differences between parts of the world and between children and adults) accept them so poorly that they must be administered via a nasogastric tube. To overcome this main constraint, the idea of the use of partial enteral nutrition (PEN) instead of EEN has emerged. Compliance and adherence to enteral nutrition would likely be much better if patients could consume some ordinary food besides the enteral formula, either unrestricted or in a form of specified elimination diets (ED). The ideal candidates for PEN are therefore all patients who are not adherent to EEN and those who do not want to receive CS due to their several side effects. In addition, there is a growing body of research addressing the possibility of nutritional treatment of CD with diets containing only a limited selection of ordinary foods without the addition of enteral formulas. Although there are many such diets, objective data on their effectiveness are very limited.

Therefore, we limited our systematic review to the efficacy of therapeutic approaches using PEN in combination with either unrestricted or specified ED for induction of CD remission in adults and children, while other nutritional treatment options are presented only in the outline of the discussion.

2. Literature search

A systematic literature search was conducted using PubMed Library on April 3, 2020. The following user query was used: ("crohn disease"[MeSH Terms] OR "crohn"[Title/Abstract] OR "crohn disease"[Title/Abstract] OR "crohn's"[Title/Abstract] OR "crohn's disease"[Title/Abstract]) AND ("enteral nutrition"[MeSH Terms] OR "enteral"[Title/Abstract] OR "enteral nutrition"[Title/Abstract]) NOT "parenteral"[Title/Abstract] NOT "exclusive"[Title/Abstract] AND "english"[language].

Based on these criteria, from 399 publications identified in PubMed database using these terms, 13 key articles were selected for further analysis, first identified study being published in 1996 (only 3 articles were published before 2004). All selected articles are gathered in **Table 1**.

Ref.	Year	Country	Type of study	n	Number of patients on PEN and comparators	Route of PEN	Type of PEN	Volume taken	Remission or relapse rates (n, %)	Significant difference (P value)
ADULT STUDIES										
Verma et al. [38]	2000	UK	Prospective non-randomised cohort study	39	PEN 21 Non-PEN 18	oral	Elemental	35–50% EAR	Remission rate at 1 year: PEN 10/21 (48%) NT 4/18 (22%)	PEN vs. non-PEN: P = 0.0003
Verma et al. [39]	2001	UK	RCT	33	ED 19 PD 14	oral	Elemental / polymeric	35–50% EAR	Remission rate at 1 year: PEN 8/19 (42%) NT 6/14 (43%)	Polymeric vs. Elemental: NS
Takagi et al. [67]	2006	Japan	RCT	51	PEN 26 Non-PEN 25	Mainly Oral/ NG	Elemental (half-elemental diet)	900–1200 ml/kcal daily	Relapse rate after 1 year: PEN 9/26 (34.6%) NT 16/25 (64%)	PEN vs. non-PEN: P < 0.01
Yamamoto et al. [40]	2007	Japan	Prospective non-randomised	40	PEN 20 non-PEN 20	NG tube at night	Elemental + low fat diet	1200–1800 ml/kcal daily	Relapse rate after 1 year: PEN 5/20 (25%) non-PEN 13/20 (65%)	PEN vs. non-PEN: P = 0.03
Yamamoto et al. [41]	2010	Japan	Prospective non-randomised	56	PEN+IFX 32 IFX 24	NG tube at night	Elemental formula + low fat diet	1200–1500 ml/kcal daily	Remission rate after 56 weeks: IFX + PEN 25/32 (78%) IFX 16/24 (67%)	IFX + PEN vs. IFX: NS
Hirai et al. [42]	2013	Japan	Retrospective-cohort study	102	PEN+IFX 45 IFX 57	Oral	Elemental formula	>900 ml/kcal daily	Remission rate after 544.1 ± 26.5 days: IFX + PEN 31/45 (69%) IFX 33/57 (42%)	IFX + PEN vs. IFX: P = 0.009

Ref.	Year	Country	Type of study	n	Number of patients on PEN and comparators	Route of PEN	Type of PEN	Volume taken	Remission or relapse rates (n, %)	Significant difference (P value)
Hanai et al. [43]	2012	Japan	RCT	95	PEN 32 MP 30 CG 33 All groups on 5-ASA	Oral/NG	Elemental	≥900 kcal daily	Remission rate at 2 years: PEN 14/32 (46.9%) MP 17/30 (56.7%) CG 7/33 (21.2%)	PEN vs. CG: $P = 0.034$ PEN vs. MP: NS
POST-SURGERY										
Yamamoto et al. [40]	2007	Japan	Prospective, non-randomised	40	PEN 20 Non-PEN 20 Both groups on 5-ASA	NG	Elemental	1200–1800 ml/kcal daily	Relapse rate at 1 year: PEN 1 (5%) CG 7 (35%) Endoscopic relapse rate at 1 year: PEN 6 (30%) CG 14 (70%)	PEN vs. CG: $P = 0.045$ PEN vs. CG: $P = 0.027$
Yamamoto et al. [44]	2013	Japan	Prospective, non-randomised	40	PEN 20 Non-PEN 20 Both groups on 5-ASA	NG	Elemental	1200–1800 ml/kcal daily	Relapse rate during 4 years of study: PEN 6 (30%) CG 12 (60%)	PEN vs. CG: NS
PAEDIATRIC STUDIES										
Wilschanski et al. [45]	1996	Canada	Retrospective cohort study	47	PEN 28 NT 19	NG tubeNocturalenteral feeding	Semi-elemental or elemental	50–60% EAR 4 or 5 nights/ week	Relapse rate at 6 months: PEN 5/28 (18%) NT 15/19 (79%) Relapse rate at 12 months: PEN 12/28 (43%) NT 15/19 (79%)	At 6 months: PEN vs. NT: $P < 0.001$ At 12 months: PEN vs. NT: $P < 0.02$

Ref.	Year	Country	Type of study	n	Number of patients on PEN and comparators	Route of PEN	Type of PEN	Volume taken	Remission or relapse rates (n, %)	Significant difference (P value)
Knight et al. [46]	2005	UK	Retrospective cohort study	40	PEN 22 NT 18	oral	Elemental or polymeric	1000 ml daily	Relapse rate at a median time of 54.5 weeks: PEN 13/22 (60%) NT 12/18 (67%)	PEN vs. NT: NS
Duncan et al. [47]	2014	UK	Retrospective cohort study	48	PEN 15 NT 13 AZA 20	Oral 14/ /NG 1	Polymeric	25% of pts. original EEN volume	PEN 9/15 (60%) NT 2/13 (15%) AZA 13/20 (65%)	PEN vs. NT: P = 0.001 PEN vs. AZA: NS
Gavin et al. [48]	2018	UK	Retrospective	102	PEN 58 NT 44	Oral	Polymeric and Elemental formula	median 30% EAR daily (range 13–65% EAR)	Relapse rate at 6 months: PEN 21/58 (36%) NT 21/44 (48%) Relapse rate within 12 months: PEN 45/58 (78%) NT 34/44 (77%) Relapse rate < 6 months EEN/PEN 14/43 (33%) CS/NT 16/29 (55%)	PEN vs. NT at 6 months: NS PEN vs. NT at 12 months: NS EEN/PEN vs. CS/NT:NS (P = 0.09)

RCT: randomised controlled trial; NS: not significant; EAR: Estimated Average Requirement; PEN: partial enteral nutrition; Non-PEN: without PEN; NT: no treatment; ED: elemental diet; PD: polymeric diet; HED: half elemental diet; MP: mercaptopurine; EEN/PEN: PEN after EEN treatment; CS/NT: no treatment (normal diet) after CS; AZA: azathioprine; CG: control group; IFX: infliximab; 5-ASA: 5-aminosalicyilic acid.

Table 1.
Summary of key studies on efficacy of partial enteral nutrition (PEN) in maintaining Crohn's disease (CD) remission.

3. Results

3.1 Partial enteral nutrition (PEN) for induction of remission in active Chron's disease (CD)

Through a systematic search, we identified 8 original articles on the use of PEN for induction of remission in active CD (**Table 1**). Of these, 5 papers presented the results of prospective controlled trials, 2 randomised and 3 non-randomised, while 3 papers described retrospective analyses of medical records of patient series. Beside to the basic methodology, research differed most in how much of a daily energy requirements patient received in the form of PEN and what they enjoyed as the rest of their daily energy requirements, unrestricted diet or special ED. In addition, we found 3 original studies using PEN simultaneously with different medical therapies for induction of remission [49–51]. It was impossible to determine how much of the effect on a disease activity could be attributed to the PEN itself from the result of these studies, so we did not include them in this review.

In 2006, Johnson et al. [52] published the results of the first prospective randomised controlled trial on the efficacy of PEN compared with EEN in inducing remission in active CD. Fifty children with active CD were randomised into two groups. In the "PEN group", children received 50% of their daily energy requirements from the elemental formula and 50% from an unrestricted diet. The control group consisted of children, treated with EEN, with 100% of their daily energy requirements provided from the elemental enteral formula. The remission rate after a 6 week-treatment period was significantly higher in EEN group (10/24, 42%) compared to the PEN group (4/26, 15%) ($P = 0.035$), pointing to a low efficacy of PEN [52]. Of note, the intention to treat remission rate in this study using elemental enteral formula was surprisingly low, even for EEN control group, in compare to majority of other studies.

In a retrospective cohort study by Gupta et al. [53] from the Children's Hospital of Philadelphia (CHOP), the remission and response rates were determined in 43 children who were treated for active CD with PEN according to the CHOP protocol, where all patients received 80–90% of their daily energy requirements from the enteral formula (elemental, semi-elemental or polymeric) and the rest from an unrestricted diet. This study showed a remission and response rate of 65% and 87%, respectively, after a mean treatment period of 2 months (1–4 months) [53]. These results are in line with the remission rates of EEN treatment reported from literature [12, 22, 54, 55]. Additionally, the study protocol with PEN was able to increase weight and improve laboratory markers in children with CD. The authors concluded that CHOP protocol, that allows patients to consume a small amount of ordinary food, has an important positive impact on treatment adherence and on the quality of life during the treatment period [53].

In a prospective cohort study, Lee et al. [56] compared clinical outcomes and mucosal healing as estimated by faecal calprotectin in 90 children with active CD receiving either PEN ($n = 16$), EEN ($n = 22$) or anti-tumour necrosis factor (TNF) therapy ($n = 52$) for induction of remission. After an 8-week treatment period, clinical response was demonstrated in 64% of patients on PEN, 88% on EEN, and 84% on anti-TNF ($P = 0.08$). EEN and anti-TNF were significantly more effective in diminishing mucosal inflammation compared to PEN. The reduction of faecal calprotectin to ≤250 μg/g was found in 14% of patients on PEN, 45% on EEN, and 62% on anti-TNF ($P < 0.001$) [56].

Wall et al. [57] performed a prospective non-randomised study including 38 adolescent and young adult patients with active CD. All patients were treated with EEN for the first two weeks, six (16%) of them discontinued this treatment in a few days because of personal decision or intolerance to polymeric enteral formula. After this initial period 21 patients were treated with EEN and 11 patients with PEN allowing one meal of ordinary food per day for another 6 weeks. Seven (33%) patients from EEN group and 2 (18%) patients from PEN did not complete the treatment, predominantly because of complications and worsening of disease. There was no significant difference between the groups ($P = 0.5$). During the initial two weeks of treatment with EEN, clinical Harvey–Bradshaw Index (HBI), serum C-reactive protein (CRP) and faecal calprotectin concentrations significantly decreased ($P = 0.003$; $P = 0.005$, $P = 0.028$). The authors observed further clinical improvement in patients who continued with EEN with significant decrease of HBI ($P = 0.031$), while markers of inflammation remained stable. In the PEN group, clinical condition and markers of inflammation did not significantly change during 6-week therapy. The authors concluded that there were no significant differences in disease activity or inflammatory markers at week 8 between patients who used EEN for 8 weeks compared with patients who used 2 weeks of EEN followed by 6 weeks of PEN [57].

In contrast with aforementioned studies allowing to eat a certain proportion of unrestricted ordinary food along with enteral formulas, other researchers combined PEN with specially designed diets.

A group of investigators from Israel led by Arie Levine developed a special diet named Crohn's disease elimination diet (CDED), based on the exclusion of dietary components hypothesised to affect either the microbiome, intestinal permeability, or innate immune system involved in CD pathogenesis. It excludes animal fats, milk and dairy, gluten and all processed and canned foods that contain additives (especially emulsifiers and maltodextrin) [58–60]. According to the authors' hypothesis, the major mechanism leading to response to EEN, is the exclusion of specific deleterious dietary factors which may impair the barrier function of the intestinal mucus layer and epithelium that allows adherence and invasion of non-pathogenic bacteria or bacterial antigens. The adherence of bacteria to the intestinal epithelium, their penetration and replication within the cells of the innate immune system such as epithelial cells, macrophages and dendritic cells can lead to continuous triggering of the adaptive immune system and therefore to the chronic inflammation [59, 61].

In 2014 the group published a retrospective report on cohort of children ($n = 34$) and young adults ($n = 13$) with active mild to moderate luminal CD who had been treated with their PEN protocol for 12 weeks. The protocol consisted of two stages. During the first 6 weeks, CDED was more restrictive and 50% of the daily energy requirements was provided in the form of polymeric enteral formula. In the second 6-week period, polymeric enteral formula was continued to supply only 25% of daily energy requirements, while small amounts of whole grain bread, and free intake of nuts, fruits, and vegetables were allowed. By week 6, a remission and response rate were 70.2% and 78.7%, respectively. The remission rates were similar in children and adults. In paediatric patients mean Paediatrics Crohn's Disease Activity Index decreased from 27.7 ± 9.4 to 5.4 ± 8.0 ($P < 0.001$). Similarly, HBI decreased from 6.4 ± 2.7 to 1.9 ± 2.9 in adults ($P < 0.001$). At week 12, 27/32 (84%) patients, that were in remission at week 6, were still in remission after the step-down phase. Normalisation in CRP was observed in 21/30 (70%) patients. Surprisingly, 6/7 (86%) patients who were treated with only CDED, without additional enteral formula, achieved remission as well [58].

In another retrospective analysis, same group reported their experience with 21 patients (11 adults and 10 children) who had lost response to biologic drugs despite dose escalation or combination therapy and were treated with PEN by a polymeric enteral formula and the CDED, 50% of daily energy requirements from each, for the first 6 weeks, followed by 6-week step-down phase as described above.

Paediatric patients with severe flares received 2 weeks of EEN followed by PEN and CDED. Clinical response was obtained in 19/21 (90.4%) patients, and remission in 13/21 (62%). Mean HBI decreased from 9.4 ± 4.2 to 2.6 ± 3.8 ($P < 0.001$). Three out of the four (75%) patients who used the CDED alone without any enteral formula supplementation, entered clinical remission. Significant decrease in CRP ($P < 0.001$) and increase in albumin concentrations ($P < 0.005$) were observed. The authors concluded that dietary treatment combining PEN and CDED may be a useful salvage regimen in CD patients failing biological therapy [62].

In 2019, Levine et al. [63] published the results of the multicentre prospective randomised controlled trial comparing the efficacy of standard EEN with CDED coupled with PEN for the induction of remission of CD. Seventy-eight children with mild to moderate active luminal CD were randomised either to EEN for 6 weeks followed by 25% of daily energy requirements intake with PEN and gradual introduction of ordinary foods during next 6 weeks or to CDED 50% and PEN 50% for the first 6 weeks followed by step-down phase CDED 75% (as explained before) with PEN 25% for the second 6 weeks. The primary endpoint of the study was patients' tolerance to both treatment regimens. The secondary endpoints were clinical response, normalisation of laboratory markers, including calprotectin as a surrogate marker for mucosal inflammation and changes in faecal microbiota. The combination of CDED and PEN was tolerated by significantly more participants (97.5%) than EEN (73.6%) ($P = 0.002$). At week 6, the remission rate in both groups did not differ significantly ($P = 0.38$). Thirty of 40 (75%) patients treated by CDEC and PEN achieved remission in compare with 20/38 (59%) treated by EEN. However, at week 12, significantly more patients given CDED and PEN group (75.6%) were in remission compared with children given EEN and then PEN without dietary restrictions (45.1%) ($P = 0.01$) [63].

Recently, Urlep et al. [64] published a prospective cohort study on efficacy of PEN combined with ED, a diet resembling CDED and based on basic foods, compared with EEN for inducing a remission in children with active CD. Twenty-five patients were allocated to a 6-week nutritional therapy with either EEN or PEN combined with one meal per day consisted of food from ED (approximately 25% of daily energy requirements). In addition to clinical evaluation and laboratory tests, ileocolonoscopy was performed before and after 6 weeks of treatment to directly assess the mucosal inflammation by using Simple Endoscopic Score (SES-CD). Clinical remission rates were similar in EEN and PEN with ED group (69,2% and 75%, respectively; $P = 0.999$). The endoscopic remission rates were 45.5% in both groups, and mucosal healing rates were also 45.5% in EEN group and 27.3% in PEN with ED group ($P = 0.659$). The study revealed that PEN in combination with relatively easy-to-keep ED was as effective as EEN for induction of both clinical and endoscopic remission [64]. However, current ECCO/ESPGHAN guidelines on medical management of paediatric CD do not recommend using PEN for the induction of remission [22].

3.2 Partial enteral nutrition (PEN) as maintenance therapy in Chron's disease (CD)

Summary of key studies on efficacy of PEN in maintaining CD remission in adult and paediatric CD patients is presented in **Table 1**.

3.2.1 PEN for maintenance therapy in adult CD

Already, in the year 1983, Harries et al. [65] reported a beneficial effect of additional enteral supplementation on the maintenance of CD remission. They conducted a controlled cross-over study in a cohort of 28 malnourished adult CD patients. For a two-month period (control period) the patients were on an unrestricted diet and for the next two-month period they received supplementary polymeric enteral formula (treatment period). The study demonstrated that the addition of enteral formula had a beneficial effect not only on the nutritional status, but also on the disease activity [65].

Ten years later, Hirakawa et al. [66] conducted a prospective controlled study in 61 CD patients who achieved remission with EEN. They were divided into 4 groups and followed-up for 1, 2 and 4 years. For maintenance of remission the first group of patients was receiving PEN in a form of elemental enteral formula in addition to their unrestricted diet. In the second group the same nutritional regimen was combined with standard medications. In the third group, only medical therapy was used, while the fourth group stayed on an unrestricted diet and without any medicines. The cumulative remission rates after 1, 2, and 4 years were significantly better in the elemental hyperalimentation group, compared with all other groups. It was concluded, that therapy with enteral nutrition has a role not only in inducing remission, but also for the maintenance of remission in CD patients [66].

In a non-randomised cohort study by Verma et al. [38], PEN was found to be more effective than an unrestricted diet for remission maintenance at 1-year follow-up. Adult patients with CD remission (n = 39) were divided into two groups according to their choice. Twenty-one out of 39 patients received elemental enteral formula (35–50% of daily energy requirements) in addition to their unrestricted diet, while the remaining 18 patients chose to have an unrestricted diet. On an intention to treat basis, 10 patients (48%) in the first group and 4 patients (22%) in the second group were still in remission at 12 months of follow-up ($P < 0.000$) [38].

In 2001, the same authors studied 33 CD patients with CS-dependent disease who were all in remission at the start of the study. They all received enteral formula in an amount that provided 35–50% of their daily energy requirements. Patients were randomised to receive either an elemental formula (n = 19) or a polymeric formula (n = 14) and were followed up for 12 months. Failure of maintenance therapy was defined by an increase in the Crohn's Disease Activity Index, inability to cessate CS or the need for surgery. According to the per-protocol data analysis, the success rate of PEN in CS-dependent patients was 14/27 (52%). The response was not significantly different between elemental (42%) and polymeric (43%) groups [39].

In a study by Takagi et al. [67], CD patients in remission, achieved with different treatment modalities (with CS, 6–8 weeks EEN, surgery, infliximab (IFX)), were randomly assigned to two groups. In the "half elemental diet group« (n = 26) patients received half of their daily energy requirements from an elemental enteral formula (900–1200 ml daily) and half from an unrestricted diet. Patients in the second group (n = 25) were on an unrestricted diet. The relapse rate was significantly lower in the half elemental group (9/26; 34.6%) in comparison with the unrestricted diet group (16/25; 64%) ($P < 0.01$), after a mean follow-up of 11.9 months. According to the results of this randomised controlled trial, with a low risk of bias, PEN seems to be a promising maintenance therapy in CD [67].

In 2006 Esaki et al. [68], conduct a retrospective study which was designed to determine risk factors for recurrence of CD under enteral nutrition. They include 145 patients with CD, who were primarily induced into remission by total parenteral nutrition. The patients were classified into two groups: enteral nutrition group (n = 98; 1200 kcal/day of enteral nutrition), or non-enteral nutrition group (n = 47; < 1200 kcal/day of enteral nutrition) according to the amount of their daily elemental or polymeric diet. Contributions of enteral nutrition and other clinical variables to the recurrence were analysed retrospectively. They conclude that among patients with CD under maintenance enteral nutrition, the risk of recurrence differs according to the disease type and the site of involvement. The maintenance treatment by enteral nutrition alone seems insufficient for patients with penetrating type or with colonic involvement [68].

In 2007 Yamamoto et al. [40] confirmed the positive impact of PEN in maintaining CD remission. They conducted a prospective controlled non-randomised study in 40 CD patients in remission. Patients in the enteral nutrition group (EN group; n = 25) received elemental enteral formula (1200–1800 ml daily) via a nasogastric tube at night and a low-fat diet during the day. Non-EN group (n = 20) was on an unrestricted diet. On an intention to treat basis, 5 patients (25%) in the EN group and 13 patients (65%) in the non-EN group relapsed during the 1-year follow-up period (P = 0.03). Furthermore, they demonstrated that the mucosal tissue levels of interleukin (IL) 1 beta, IL-6 and TNF-alpha significantly increased in the non-EN group during 1 year of follow-up, while the levels of these cytokines in the EN group did not change significantly. Similarly, the mucosal inflammation seen by ileocolonoscopies was significantly increased in the non-EN group. The researchers concluded that PEN is effective in diminishing clinical relapse rates and in suppressing cytokine production and mucosal inflammation in CD patients who entered clinical remission. Limitations of the study are its relatively small number of patients and a non-randomised design. Only patients with good compliance were assigned to the EN group, therefore, the bias of the study is high. Nevertheless, this study clearly shows that PEN has a positive effect not only on clinical activity but also on inflammation of the gut mucosa [40].

In 2009, Takagi et al. [69] investigated the quality of life of patients on PEN for maintenance of remission and the medical cost of this treatment regimen. This is an extension study of their previous randomised controlled trial [67], which showed that quality of life did not significantly differ between the two groups of patients; the PEN and the non-PEN group. Interestingly, there was also no statistically significant difference in the medical costs between these two groups of CD patients [69].

Yamamoto et al. [41] conducted a prospective study to examine the efficacy of combined PEN and IFX maintenance treatment. Patients who achieved remission with IFX and were treated with regular IFX infusions to maintain remission (5 mg/kg every 8 weeks) were divided into two groups. In the first group patients received IFX with concomitant PEN (1200–1500 ml of elemental enteral formula at night and low-fat diet during the day). The second group was treated only with maintenance IFX without PEN. Surprisingly, there was no statistically significant difference observed in remission rates between the two groups at the end of the 56-week follow-up (P = 0.51) [41]. However, this study was not randomised, and it involved only a small cohort of patients.

On the contrary, other studies demonstrated the beneficial effect of combined PEN and IFX maintenance treatment. In a retrospective study by Hirai et al. [42], 45 patients on maintenance therapy with IFX received concomitant PEN (elemental formula; > 900 kcal daily) and 57 patients were administered only IFX without PEN. The patients were followed for 544 ± 27 days. The cumulative remission rate was significantly higher in the combined PEN and IFX group in comparison to the non-combined group (P = 0.009) [42]. The authors hypothesised that PEN contributed to the positive effect of maintenance IFX due to its anti-inflammatory effect [70–73], the effect on cytokine production and the beneficial effect on gut microbiota [74–77].

Similar findings were observed in a multicentric retrospective study by Kamata et al. [78]. They found that concomitant PEN (≥ 900 kcal daily) during IFX maintenance therapy significantly prolonged the remission period. The group of CD patients treated with combined PEN and IFX therapy showed significantly lower cumulative loss of response rate in comparison with the non-combined group ($P < 0.049$). The authors believe that PEN may decrease intestinal inflammation, therefore less serum IFX levels may be effective for controlling the disease [78].

In a meta-analysis by Nguyen et al. [79], the effect of concomitant PEN therapy with IFX in comparison with IFX monotherapy was assessed for maintenance of CD remission. Four studies met the inclusion criteria [41, 42, 80, 81]. In the group of patients on the combined PEN and IFX therapy, significantly higher percentage of patients (74.5%) remained in clinical remission in comparison with the IFX monotherapy group (49.2%) after 1 year of follow-up period ($P < 0.01$) [79].

Hanai et al. [43] conducted the only adult randomised controlled study comparing the efficacy of PEN with 6-mercaptopurine (6-MP) in maintaining CD remission. They studied 95 patients with CD in remission who were split into 3 groups. All patients took 5-aminosalicylic acid (2250–3000 mg per day). In the first group ($n = 30$) they received 6-MP (0.5–1.5 mg/day), in the second group ($n = 32$) they were on PEN (elemental enteral formula; ≥ 900 kcal daily and intake of 3.5–4.0 kcal/kg/day from food in line with the recommendation of a qualified dietician), in the third group ($n = 33$) patients received only 5-aminosalicylic acid (control group). The percentage of patients who were still in remission after 2 years of follow-up were 56.7% (MP group), 46.9% (PEN group) and 21.2% (control group), respectively. There was a significantly higher remission rate in the PEN group versus the control group ($P < 0.034$). Furthermore, the remission rates between PEN and MP group did not differ significantly ($P = 0.273$) [43]. Although this is a prospective randomised controlled study, its limitation is relatively small sample size. Therefore, further larger studies should be conducted to confirm these results. As thiopurines are drugs with many side effects [82], results of such studies would be desirable to decide upon an appropriate maintenance therapy, that should have a high ratio between efficiency and adverse effects.

3.2.2 PEN for maintenance therapy after surgery in CD patients

Some smaller retrospective studies demonstrated that therapy with enteral nutrition had reduced relapse rate after surgery in CD patients [83, 84].

In Ikeuchi et al. [83], they examined the effects of postoperative nutritional therapy in patients with perforating and non-perforating type of CD. They retrospectively reviewed the records for 218 patients who underwent surgical interventions for CD between 1974 and 2001. Patients were divided into four groups: 92 patients in the non-perforating type group had received an elemental diet, 22 patients in the non-perforating type had received an unrestricted diet, 88 patients in the perforating type had received an elemental diet and 16 patients in perforated type had received an unrestricted diet. They conclude that in patients with CD postoperative elemental diet and nutritional education is effective in reducing the incidence of second resection. It appears that postoperative elemental diet and nutritional education is more important in patients with perforated type CD [83].

Therefore, Yamamoto et al. [85] conducted the first prospective non-randomised study in 40 consecutive adult patients after resection for ileal or ileocolonic CD. Patients were assigned either to the PEN group ($n = 20$) or to the control group ($n = 20$) with an unrestricted diet. In the PEN group, patients received elemental enteral formula (1200–1800 ml daily) at night, through a nasogastric tube, and a low-fat diet during the day. Patients from both groups additionally took 5-aminosalicyilic acid 3000 mg daily. Ileocolonoscopy was performed at 6 and 12 months after surgery. One patient from the PEN group (5%) and 7 patients (35%) from the control group relapsed during the 1-year follow-up period ($P = 0.048$). Furthermore,

6 patients (30%) in the PEN group and 14 patients (70%) in the control group developed endoscopic recurrence by 12 months after surgery (P = 0.027) [85].

In 2013 the same authors published an extension study on the long-term efficacy of PEN as a maintenance therapy in CD patients who underwent surgery. Twenty patients were on PEN, delivered as a continuous elemental enteral formula during the night-time, and on a low-fat diet during the day. Twenty control group CD patients were given an unrestricted diet without therapy until disease recurrence. Recurrence rates after 5-year-follow-up were significantly lower in the PEN group compared to the control group (P = 0.02). This study confirmed the results of the previous study and showed that PEN may be effective in maintaining remission in CD patients after surgery [44]. However, both studies included a small number of patients and only the highly compliant ones were assigned to PEN group, so the risk of bias was high.

3.2.3 PEN for maintenance therapy in paediatric CD patients

In 1982 Navarro et al. [86] first reported the use of prolonged constant rate elemental enteral nutrition (CREN) in CD. It has been used in 17 paediatric patients with CD. Exclusive CREN was maintained from 2 to 7 months and progressively reduced to assure fractioned oral intakes from 12 to 22 months. From this preliminary study, CREN appeared to be as effective as CS therapy in initiating remission of active CD and was able to supress CS dependence. In some cases, with prolonged CREN, reduction or disappearance of stenotic lesions of the bowel was observed. Two other positive points must be emphasised: the favourable psychological impact of the method and the ability to avoid growth suppression secondary to CS. The long-term effects and longer remission must be confirmed by a multicentre study in a larger group of patients [86].

In 1988 Belli et al. [87] demonstrated decreased activity of CD and improvement in growth in a group of 8 children who had received elemental enteral formula at cyclical periods of time (one out of 4 months) for 1 year [87]. Although this was a small study, it encouraged further investigations on maintenance therapy with enteral nutrition.

Wilschanski et al. [45] conducted a retrospective study on 47 children and adolescents with CD who achieved clinical remission after EEN induction therapy. Twenty-eight patients continued with nocturnal PEN through a nasogastric tube and 19 patients consumed an unrestricted diet without enteral supplementation. The relapse rate was significantly higher in patients on an unrestricted diet in comparison with those who were treated with PEN at 6 (P < 0.001) and 12 months (P < 0.02), respectively. Furthermore, the group of patients on nocturnal PEN who had not yet completed puberty had improved linear growth compared to similar patients who were on an unrestricted diet [45].

On the contrary, Knight et al. [46] did not confirm the better outcome in patients receiving PEN. They retrospectively studied the short and long-term outcomes of using enteral nutrition for induction and maintenance of remission in paediatric CD patients. Out of 79 newly diagnosed CD patients, 44 (55%) chose EEN as the primary induction therapy and 40 (90%) of those responded to treatment. These 40 patients were then encouraged to continue with maintenance PEN (1000 ml of elemental or polymeric enteral formula daily) in addition to an unrestricted diet, but only 22 (55%) were able to accept the PEN treatment protocol. The authors did not find a statistically significant difference in the remission rates between the two groups [46]. However, the consumed volume of enteral formula was not carefully recorded, this could have affected the results and may have led to the higher rate of treatment failure [46].

A study by Duncan et al. [47] showed completely opposite results. In this retrospective study, 48 CD patients who entered clinical remission or responded to an eight-week treatment with EEN, were encouraged to continue a maintenance therapy with 25% of the volume of the previously used elemental or polymeric enteral formula. Only 15 out of 48 (31%) patients chose PEN, for a mean time of 11 months (range 4–14 months). Twenty (42%) patients took azathioprine and 13 (27%) patients had no maintenance treatment. Remission rates at one year were 60% in the PEN group, 65% in the azathioprine group and 15% in the control group. There was a significantly higher remission rate in the PEN group versus the control group ($P = 0.001$). Furthermore, remission rates between PEN and azathioprine group were not significantly different ($P = 0.14$) [47].

In 2015 Konno et al. [88], reported their real-life data on the long-term outcome of maintenance treatment with PEN in a consecutive cohort of 58 paediatric CD patients who entered remission with different treatment regimens. All 58 patients received PEN with a least 30 kcal/kg/day of elemental enteral formula in conjunction with a low-fat diet (< 20 g fat/day). In addition, they were treated only with 5-ASA, until first relapse. Fifty-two out of 58 patients took enteral formula orally and the remaining 6 through a nasogastric tube. The relapse rates were 12% at 1 year, 27% at 2 years, and 48% at 5 years, respectively [88]. This study surprisingly showed that approximately half of the children who received PEN as a maintenance therapy were able to sustain remission for 5 years without taking other medication such as immunosuppressives.

Schulman et al. [89] studied 42 CD paediatric patients who entered clinical remission after EEN and received PEN as a supplementary diet (50% of daily energy requirements as polymeric enteral formula). The control group consisted of patients who refused PEN. They found that the total increase in body mass index (BMI) and the total decrease in the mean weighted Paediatric Crohn's Disease Activity Index between the time of diagnosis and eight months after diagnosis were greater in the PEN group compared to the control group. Furthermore, in the PEN group there was better improvement in albumin and CRP levels in comparison with the control group. However, more than 50% of patients required concomitant maintenance therapy within two weeks of PEN initiation and most of patients required concomitant immunosuppressive therapy at some point after initiation of PEN [89].

Gavin et al. [48], reported real-life data on their experience with EEN as induction therapy and PEN as a maintenance therapy. 102 newly diagnosed paediatric CD patients were included. Seventy-seven (75%) patients were treated with a 6–8-week course of EEN and the remaining 25 with CS (25%). The remission rate in the EEN group was 76% and in the CS group 75% respectively. Following induction treatment, 58 out of 102 (57%) patients received PEN as a maintenance therapy (median 30% of daily energy needs; range from 13 to 65% of daily energy requirements of polymeric or elemental formula) and rest as an unrestricted diet. Forty-four out of 102 (43%) patients consumed an unrestricted diet for a median duration of 4 months (range 1–12 months). The increase of BMI z-score was significantly higher in the PEN group in comparison with the unrestricted diet group. However, relapse rates were similar in both groups at 6 and 12 months [48].

El-Matary et al. [90], published a systematic review on the efficacy of maintenance PEN. Databases were searched to April 2015. Twelve studies met the inclusion criteria; however, a meta-analysis was not performed due to the excessive heterogeneity of the studies. Out of these 12 studies, 11 of them had shown a beneficial effect of PEN in maintaining remission, therefore, authors concluded that PEN was more effective than unrestricted diet in maintaining CD remission [90].

Gavin et al. [91] conduct a survey including patients, parents and UK dietitians regarding their experience with maintenance enteral nutrition (MEN) which is often routinely used in paediatric CD to prolong remission although there is limited evidence for efficacy and a lack of formal guidelines. They identified a different perspective between patients, families and professionals on the use of MEN. Young people and parents reported difficulties with adherence to MEN especially due to the taste and they stated a preference for dietary advice. This study advocates that the extensive use of MEN in clinical practice is limited to comply with ESPGHAN recommendations. Patient led care promotes the use of dietary advice as a mode of nutritional support during inactive disease [91].

In Kim et al. study [92], they determine the abilities of EEN and PEN to induce and maintain clinical remission in paediatric patients with CD, respectively. All paediatric patients with CD who received EEN at a single centre in 2000–2014 were identified retrospectively. Remission rates of the EEN and PEN during the 2 years study period were determined. Risk factors for EEN and PEN failure were also identified. They conclude that EEN and PEN effectively induced and maintained remission in a paediatric population. However, non-adherence was a limiting factor in the success of therapy, especially in females [92].

In Watanabe et al. [93], they investigate the effectiveness of enteral nutrition with an elemental diet regarding the avoidance of hospitalisation. Altogether 268 patients with CD who visited hospital from 2003 to 2008 were enrolled. The relationship between the proportion of energy consumed with an elemental diet and hospitalisation as an endpoint was examined retrospectively. They conclude that the use of an elemental diet of 900 kcal/day may be effective in avoiding hospitalisation in CD patients with ileal lesions. However, this diet may be useful in improving the long-term convalescence of these patients [93].

According to the current ECCO/ESPGHAN clinical guidelines on CD, in children with low-risk CD who achieved clinical remission, monotherapy with maintenance enteral nutrition (at least 50% of daily energy requirements) can prolong remission [22].

4. Conclusions

Despite the evidence that EEN is an effective and safe therapeutic option in inducing remission in paediatric and potentially in adult active CD and it is substantially more effective in promoting mucosal healing compared to CS, it is still underused in clinical practice. Its biggest disadvantage is patients' compliance. Taste fatigue due to the poor palatability and the subsequent negative impact on the quality of life remain the most important reasons why EEN therapy is not acceptable to many patients. Thus, the use of PEN, where some ordinary food, besides enteral formulas, can be consumed, is rapidly becoming an interesting therapeutic option. Unfortunately, the first well designed, prospective randomised controlled trial on PEN did not confirm PEN efficacy in inducing remission in active CD [52]. However, some recent small and retrospective studies pointed to the possible beneficial effect of PEN in active CD. Larger prospective randomised studies are needed to examine the possible role of PEN in inducing remission in paediatric and adult CD.

While EEN is not an acceptable therapeutic option for maintenance of CD remission in clinical practice, several studies examined the efficacy and the usefulness of PEN in maintaining remission in adult and paediatric CD (**Table 1**). The results were conflicting. Most of these studies were non-randomised, with only a small number of patients included. However, the results of some recent studies, including the Japanese randomised controlled trials with a large enough sample size and a sufficiently low risk of bias [67], were promising and indicated that PEN might be effective in maintaining CD remission.

Due to the excellent safety profile of enteral nutrition, treatment with PEN in inducing and maintaining remission in CD patients merits further investigation. Larger, well-designed, randomised controlled studies on the efficacy of PEN as a monotherapy or in combination with other medications and/or ED are needed in adults and the paediatric CD population.

Conflict of interest

The authors declare no conflict of interest.

Author details

Evgen Benedik[1,2]*, Darja Urlep[1], Anija Orel[1,3] and Rok Orel[1]

1 Division of Paediatrics, Department of Gastroenterology, Hepatology and Nutrition, University Medical Centre Ljubljana, Ljubljana, Slovenia

2 Human Nutrition Group, Department of Food Science and Technology, Biotechnical Faculty, University of Ljubljana, Ljubljana, Slovenia

3 Division of Paediatrics, Unit of Diet Therapy and Hospital Nutrition Care Services, University Medical Centre Ljubljana, Ljubljana, Slovenia

*Address all correspondence to: evgen.benedik@kclj.si

References

[1] Jantchou P, Morois S, Clavel-Chapelon F, Boutron-Ruault M-C, Carbonnel F. Animal protein intake and risk of inflammatory bowel disease: The E3N prospective study. Am J Gastroenterol. 2010 Oct;105(10):2195-201.

[2] Hou JK, Abraham B, El-Serag H. Dietary intake and risk of developing inflammatory bowel disease: a systematic review of the literature. Am J Gastroenterol. 2011 Apr;106(4):563-73.

[3] Ananthakrishnan AN, Khalili H, Konijeti GG, Higuchi LM, de Silva P, Korzenik JR, et al. A prospective study of long-term intake of dietary fiber and risk of Crohn's disease and ulcerative colitis. Gastroenterology. 2013 Nov;145(5):970-7.

[4] Ananthakrishnan AN, Khalili H, Konijeti GG, Higuchi LM, de Silva P, Fuchs CS, et al. Long-term intake of dietary fat and risk of ulcerative colitis and Crohn's disease. Gut [Internet]. 2014 May [cited 2014 Jul 28];63(5):776-84. Available from: http://www.ncbi.nlm.nih.gov/pubmed/23828881

[5] Conrad MA, Rosh JR. Pediatric Inflammatory Bowel Disease. Pediatr Clin North Am. 2017 Jun;64(3):577-91.

[6] Kotlyar DS, Lewis JD, Beaugerie L, Tierney A, Brensinger CM, Gisbert JP, et al. Risk of Lymphoma in Patients With Inflammatory Bowel Disease Treated With Azathioprine and 6-Mercaptopurine: A Meta-analysis. Clin Gastroenterol Hepatol. 2015 May;13(5):847-858.e4.

[7] Dulai PS, Thompson KD, Blunt HB, Dubinsky MC, Siegel CA. Risks of Serious Infection or Lymphoma With Anti–Tumor Necrosis Factor Therapy for Pediatric Inflammatory Bowel Disease: A Systematic Review. Clin Gastroenterol Hepatol. 2014 Sep;12(9):1443-51.

[8] Garg SK, Velayos FS, Kisiel JB. Intestinal and Nonintestinal Cancer Risks for Patients with Crohn's Disease. Gastroenterol Clin North Am. 2017 Sep;46(3):515-29.

[9] Kruis W, Nguyen PG, Morgenstern J. Promises and Dangers of Combination Therapy. Dig Dis. 2017;35(1-2):56-60.

[10] Heuschkel RB, Menache CC, Megerian JT, Baird AE. Enteral nutrition and corticosteroids in the treatment of acute Crohn's disease in children. J Pediatr Gastroenterol Nutr. 2000 Jul;31(1):8-15.

[11] Dziechciarz P, Horvath A, Shamir R, Szajewska H. Meta-analysis: enteral nutrition in active Crohn's disease in children. Aliment Pharmacol Ther. 2007 Jul 7;26(6):795-806.

[12] Swaminath A, Feathers A, Ananthakrishnan AN, Falzon L, Li Ferry S. Systematic review with meta-analysis: enteral nutrition therapy for the induction of remission in paediatric Crohn's disease. Aliment Pharmacol Ther. 2017 Oct;46(7):645-56.

[13] Zachos M, Tondeur M, Griffiths AM. Enteral nutritional therapy for induction of remission in Crohn's disease. In: Zachos M, editor. Cochrane Database of Systematic Reviews. Chichester, UK: John Wiley & Sons, Ltd; 2007. p. CD000542.

[14] Narula N, Dhillon A, Zhang D, Sherlock ME, Tondeur M, Zachos M. Enteral nutritional therapy for induction of remission in Crohn's disease. Cochrane database Syst Rev. 2018 Apr;4(4):CD000542.

[15] Yu Y, Chen K-C, Chen J. Exclusive enteral nutrition versus corticosteroids for treatment of pediatric Crohn's disease: a meta-analysis. World J Pediatr [Internet]. 2019 Feb 21 [cited

2019 Jul 2];15(1):26-36. Available from: http://www.ncbi.nlm.nih.gov/pubmed/30666565

[16] Grover Z, Muir R, Lewindon P. Exclusive enteral nutrition induces early clinical, mucosal and transmural remission in paediatric Crohn's disease. J Gastroenterol. 2014 Apr 30;49(4):638-45.

[17] Chen J-M, He L-W, Yan T, Guo X-F, Hu P-J, Peng J-S, et al. Oral exclusive enteral nutrition induces mucosal and transmural healing in patients with Crohn's disease. Gastroenterol Rep [Internet]. 2019 Jun 1;7(3):176-84. Available from: https://doi.org/10.1093/gastro/goy050

[18] Ley D, Duhamel A, Behal H, Vasseur F, Sarter H, Michaud L, et al. Growth Pattern in Paediatric Crohn Disease Is Related to Inflammatory Status. J Pediatr Gastroenterol Nutr. 2016 Dec;63(6):637-43.

[19] Shamir R, Phillip M, Levine A. Growth retardation in pediatric Crohn's disease: pathogenesis and interventions. Inflamm Bowel Dis. 2007 May;13(5):620-8.

[20] Sanderson IR. Growth problems in children with IBD. Nat Rev Gastroenterol Hepatol. 2014 Jun 24;11(10):601-10.

[21] Griffiths AM. Growth Retardation in Early-Onset Inflammatory Bowel Disease: Should We Monitor and Treat These Patients Differently? Dig Dis. 2009;27(3):404-11.

[22] van Rheenen PF, Aloi M, Assa A, Bronsky J, Escher JC, Fagerberg UL, et al. The medical management of paediatric Crohn's disease: an ECCO-ESPGHAN guideline update. J Crohns Colitis. 2020, jjaa161.

[23] O'Morain C. Elemental diets and Crohn's disease. Acta Gastroenterol Belg. 1987;50(5):574-8.

[24] Engelman J, Black L, Murphy G, Sladen G. Comparison of a semi elemental diet (Peptamen) with prednisolonin the primary-treatment of active ileal Crohn's disease. Gastroenterology. 1993;104:A697–A697.

[25] Mantzaris G, Archavlis E, Amperiadis P, Kourtessas D, Triantafyllou G. A randomized prospective trial in active Crohn's disease comparing a polymeric diet, prednisolone, and a polymeric diet plus prednisolone. Gastroenterology. 1996;110:A955–A955.

[26] Zoli G, Carè M, Parazza M, Spanò C, Biagi PL, Bernardi M, et al. A randomized controlled study comparing elemental diet and steroid treatment in Crohn's disease. Aliment Pharmacol Ther. 1997 Aug;11(4):735-40.

[27] Gassull MA, Fernández-Bañares F, Cabré E, Papo M, Giaffer MH, Sánchez-Lombraña JL, et al. Fat composition may be a clue to explain the primary therapeutic effect of enteral nutrition in Crohn's disease: results of a double blind randomised multicentre European trial. Gut. 2002 Aug;51(2):164-8.

[28] Griffiths AM, Ohlsson A, Sherman PM, Sutherland LR. Meta-analysis of enteral nutrition as a primary treatment of active Crohn's disease. Gastroenterology. 1995 Apr;108(4):1056-67.

[29] Fernández-Bañares F, Cabré E, Esteve-Comas M, Gassull MA. How Effective Is Enteral Nutrition in Inducing Clinical Remission in Active Crohn's Disease? A Meta-Analysis of the Randomized Clinical Trials. J Parenter Enter Nutr. 1995 Sep 2;19(5):356-64.

[30] Messori A, Trallori G, D'Albasio G, Milla M, Vannozzi G, Pacini F. Defined-formula diets versus steroids in the treatment of active Crohn's disease: a meta-analysis. Scand J Gastroenterol. 1996 Mar;31(3):267-72.

[31] Zachos M, Tondeur M, Griffiths A. Enteral nutritional therapy for induction of remission in Crohn's disease. In: Zachos M, editor. The Cochrane Database of Systematic Reviews. Chichester, UK: John Wiley & Sons, Ltd; 2001. p. CD000542.

[32] Durchschein F, Petritsch W, Hammer HF. Diet therapy for inflammatory bowel diseases: The established and the new. World J Gastroenterol. 2016 Feb 21;22(7):2179-94.

[33] Matsuoka K, Kobayashi T, Ueno F, Matsui T, Hirai F, Inoue N, et al. Evidence-based clinical practice guidelines for inflammatory bowel disease. J Gastroenterol [Internet]. 2018;53(3):305-53. Available from: https://doi.org/10.1007/s00535-018-1439-1

[34] Okada M, Yao T, Yamamoto T, Takenaka K, Imamura K, Maeda K, et al. Controlled trial comparing an elemental diet with prednisolone in the treatment of active Crohn's disease. Hepatogastroenterology. 1990 Feb;37(1):72-80.

[35] Gomollón F, Dignass A, Annese V, Tilg H, Van Assche G, Lindsay JO, et al. 3rd European Evidence-based Consensus on the Diagnosis and Management of Crohn's Disease 2016: Part 1: Diagnosis and Medical Management. J Crohn's Colitis [Internet]. 2017 Jan 1;11(1):3-25. Available from: https://doi.org/10.1093/ecco-jcc/jjw168

[36] Torres J, Bonovas S, Doherty G, Kucharzik T, Gisbert JP, Raine T, et al. ECCO Guidelines on Therapeutics in Crohn's Disease: Medical Treatment. J Crohn's Colitis [Internet]. 2020 Jan 1;14(1):4-22. Available from: https://doi.org/10.1093/ecco-jcc/jjz180

[37] Bischoff SC, Escher J, Hébuterne X, Kłęk S, Krznaric Z, Schneider S, et al. ESPEN practical guideline: Clinical Nutrition in inflammatory bowel disease. Clin Nutr [Internet]. 2020;39(3):632-53. Available from: http://www.sciencedirect.com/science/article/pii/S0261561419331280

[38] Verma S, Kirkwood B, Brown S, Giaffer MH. Oral nutritional supplementation is effective in the maintenance of remission in Crohn's disease. Dig Liver Dis. 2000 Dec;32(9):769-74.

[39] Verma S, Holdsworth CD, Giaffer MH. Does adjuvant nutritional support diminish steroid dependency in Crohn disease? Scand J Gastroenterol. 2001 Apr;36(4):383-8.

[40] Yamamoto T, Nakahigashi M, Saniabadi AR, Iwata T, Maruyama Y, Umegae S, et al. Impacts of long-term enteral nutrition on clinical and endoscopic disease activities and mucosal cytokines during remission in patients with Crohn's disease: A prospective study. Inflamm Bowel Dis. 2007 Dec;13(12):1493-501.

[41] Yamamoto T, Nakahigashi M, Umegae S, Matsumoto K. Prospective clinical trial: enteral nutrition during maintenance infliximab in Crohn's disease. J Gastroenterol. 2010 Jan 2;45(1):24-9.

[42] Hirai F, Ishihara H, Yada S, Esaki M, Ohwan T, Nozaki R, et al. Effectiveness of Concomitant Enteral Nutrition Therapy and Infliximab for Maintenance Treatment of Crohn's Disease in Adults. Dig Dis Sci. 2013 May 29;58(5):1329-34.

[43] Hanai H, Iida T, Takeuchi K, Arai H, Arai O, Abe J, et al. Nutritional therapy versus 6-mercaptopurine as maintenance therapy in patients with Crohn's disease. Dig Liver Dis. 2012 Aug;44(8):649-54.

[44] Yamamoto T, Shiraki M, Nakahigashi M, Umegae S, Matsumoto K. Enteral nutrition to

suppress postoperative Crohn's disease recurrence: a five-year prospective cohort study. Int J Colorectal Dis. 2013 Mar 27;28(3):335-40.

[45] Wilschanski M, Sherman P, Pencharz P, Davis L, Corey M, Griffiths A. Supplementary enteral nutrition maintains remission in paediatric Crohn's disease. Gut. 1996 Apr;38(4):543-8.

[46] Knight C, El-Matary W, Spray C, Sandhu BK. Long-term outcome of nutritional therapy in paediatric Crohn's disease. Clin Nutr. 2005 Oct;24(5):775-9.

[47] Duncan H, Buchanan E, Cardigan T, Garrick V, Curtis L, McGrogan P, et al. A retrospective study showing maintenance treatment options for paediatric CD in the first year following diagnosis after induction of remission with EEN: supplemental enteral nutrition is better than nothing! BMC Gastroenterol. 2014 Dec 20;14(1):50.

[48] Gavin J, Ashton J, Heather N, Marino L, Beattie R. Nutritional support in paediatric Crohn's disease: outcome at 12 months. Acta Paediatr. 2018 Jan;107(1):156-62.

[49] Hartman C, Berkowitz D, Weiss B, Shaoul R, Levine A, Adiv OE, et al. Nutritional Supplementation with Polymeric Diet Enriched with Transforming Growth Factor-Beta 2 for Children with Crohn ' s Disease. 2008;10(July):503-7.

[50] Kang Y, Kim S, Kim SY, Koh H. Effect of short-term partial enteral nutrition on the treatment of younger patients with severe Crohn's disease. Gut Liver [Internet]. 2015;9(1):87—93. Available from: https://europepmc.org/articles/PMC4282862

[51] Agin M, Yucel A, Gumus M, Yuksekkaya HA, Tumgor G. The Effect of Enteral Nutrition Support Rich in TGF-β in the Treatment of Inflammatory Bowel Disease in Childhood. Medicina (B Aires) [Internet]. 2019 Sep 22 [cited 2020 Oct 21];55(10):620. Available from: https://www.mdpi.com/1010-660X/55/10/620

[52] Johnson T, Macdonald S, Hill SM, Thomas A, Murphy MS. Treatment of active Crohn's disease in children using partial enteral nutrition with liquid formula: a randomised controlled trial. Gut. 2006 Mar;55(3):356-61.

[53] Gupta K, Noble A, Kachelries KE, Albenberg L, Kelsen JR, Grossman AB, et al. A novel enteral nutrition protocol for the treatment of pediatric Crohn's disease. Inflamm Bowel Dis. 2013;19(7):1374-8.

[54] Borrelli O, Cordischi L, Cirulli M, Paganelli M, Labalestra V, Uccini S, et al. Polymeric Diet Alone Versus Corticosteroids in the Treatment of Active Pediatric Crohn's Disease: A Randomized Controlled Open-Label Trial. Clin Gastroenterol Hepatol. 2006 Jun;4(6):744-53.

[55] Berni Canani R, Terrin G, Borrelli O, Romano MT, Manguso F, Coruzzo A, et al. Short- and long-term therapeutic efficacy of nutritional therapy and corticosteroids in paediatric Crohn's disease. Dig Liver Dis. 2006 Jun;38(6):381-7.

[56] Lee D, Baldassano RN, Otley AR, Albenberg L, Griffiths AM, Compher C, et al. Comparative Effectiveness of Nutritional and Biological Therapy in North American Children with Active Crohn's Disease. Inflamm Bowel Dis. 2015 Aug;21(8):1786-93.

[57] Wall CL, Gearry RB, Day AS. Treatment of Active Crohn's Disease with Exclusive and Partial Enteral Nutrition: A Pilot Study in Adults. Inflamm Intest Dis [Internet]. 2017;2(4):219-27. Available from: https://www.karger.com/DOI/10.1159/000489630

[58] Sigall-Boneh R, Pfeffer-Gik T, Segal I, Zangen T, Boaz M, Levine A. Partial Enteral Nutrition with a Crohn's Disease Exclusion Diet Is Effective for Induction of Remission in Children and Young Adults with Crohn's Disease. Inflamm Bowel Dis. 2014 Aug;20(8):1353-60.

[59] Pfeffer-Gik T, Levine A. Dietary Clues to the Pathogenesis of Crohn's Disease. Dig Dis. 2014;32(4):389-94.

[60] Levine A, Wine E. Effects of enteral nutrition on Crohn's disease: clues to the impact of diet on disease pathogenesis. Inflamm Bowel Dis. 2013 May;19(6):1322-9.

[61] Sarbagili-Shabat C, Sigall-Boneh R, Levine A. Nutritional therapy in inflammatory bowel disease. Curr Opin Gastroenterol. 2015 Jul;31(4):303-8.

[62] Sigall Boneh R, Sarbagili Shabat C, Yanai H, Chermesh I, Ben Avraham S, Boaz M, et al. Dietary Therapy With the Crohn's Disease Exclusion Diet is a Successful Strategy for Induction of Remission in Children and Adults Failing Biological Therapy. J Crohns Colitis. 2017 Oct;11(10):1205-12.

[63] Levine A, Wine E, Assa A, Sigall Boneh R, Shaoul R, Kori M, et al. Crohn's Disease Exclusion Diet Plus Partial Enteral Nutrition Induces Sustained Remission in a Randomized Controlled Trial. Gastroenterology. 2019 Aug;157(2):440-450.e8.

[64] Urlep D, Benedik E, Brecelj J, Orel R. Partial enteral nutrition induces clinical and endoscopic remission in active pediatric Crohn's disease: results of a prospective cohort study. Eur J Pediatr. 2020 Mar;179(3):431-8.

[65] Harries AD, Jones LA, Danis V, Fifield R, Heatley R V, Newcombe RG, et al. Controlled trial of supplemented oral nutrition in Crohn's disease. Lancet (London, England). 1983 Apr 23;1(8330):887-90.

[66] Hirakawa H, Fukuda Y, Tanida N, Hosomi M, Shimoyama T. Home elemental enteral hyperalimentation (HEEH) for the maintenance of remission in patients with Crohn's disease. Gastroenterol Jpn. 1993 Jun;28(3):379-84.

[67] Takagi S, Utsunomiya K, Kuriyama S, Yokoyama H, Takahashi S, Iwabuchi M, et al. Effectiveness of an "half elemental diet" as maintenance therapy for Crohn's disease: a randomized-controlled trial. Aliment Pharmacol Ther. 2006 Nov 1;24(9):1333-40.

[68] Esaki M, Matsumoto T, Nakamura S, Yada S, Fujisawa K, Jo Y, et al. Factors affecting recurrence in patients with Crohn's disease under nutritional therapy. Dis *Colon rectum*. 2006 Oct;49(10 Suppl):S68-74.

[69] Takagi S, Utsunomiya K, Kuriyama S, Yokoyama H, Takahashi S, Umemura K, et al. Quality of life of patients and medical cost of "half elemental diet" as maintenance therapy for Crohn's disease: Secondary outcomes of a randomised controlled trial. Dig Liver Dis. 2009 Jun;41(6):390-4.

[70] Fell JM, Paintin M, Arnaud-Battandier F, Beattie RM, Hollis A, Kitching P, et al. Mucosal healing and a fall in mucosal pro-inflammatory cytokine mRNA induced by a specific oral polymeric diet in paediatric Crohn's disease. Aliment Pharmacol Ther. 2000 Mar;14(3):281-9.

[71] Nahidi L, Corley SM, Wilkins MR, Wei J, Alhagamhmad M, Day AS, et al. The major pathway by which polymeric formula reduces inflammation in intestinal epithelial cells: a microarray-based analysis. Genes Nutr. 2015 Sep 17;10(5):29.

[72] Guo Z, Gong J, Li Y, Gu L, Cao L, Wang Z, et al. Mucosal MicroRNAs Expression Profiles before and after

Exclusive Enteral Nutrition Therapy in Adult Patients with Crohn's Disease. Nutrients. 2016 Aug 22;8(8):519.

[73] Budd GR, Aitchison A, Day AS, Keenan JI. The effect of polymeric formula on enterocyte differentiation. Innate Immun. 2017 Apr 19;23(3):240-8.

[74] Lionetti P, Callegari ML, Ferrari S, Cavicchi MC, Pozzi E, de Martino M, et al. Enteral Nutrition and Microflora in Pediatric Crohn's Disease. J Parenter Enter Nutr. 2005 Jul 11;29(4_suppl):S173-8.

[75] Leach ST, Mitchell HM, Eng WR, Zhang L, Day AS. Sustained modulation of intestinal bacteria by exclusive enteral nutrition used to treat children with Crohn's disease. Aliment Pharmacol Ther. 2008 Sep 15;28(6):724-33.

[76] Day AS, Lopez RN. Exclusive enteral nutrition in children with Crohn's disease. World J Gastroenterol. 2015 Jun 14;21(22):6809-16.

[77] Gerasimidis K, Bertz M, Hanske L, Junick J, Biskou O, Aguilera M, et al. Decline in Presumptively Protective Gut Bacterial Species and Metabolites Are Paradoxically Associated with Disease Improvement in Pediatric Crohn's Disease During Enteral Nutrition. Inflamm Bowel Dis. 2014 May;20(5):861-71.

[78] Kamata N, Oshitani N, Watanabe K, Watanabe K, Hosomi S, Noguchi A, et al. Efficacy of Concomitant Elemental Diet Therapy in Scheduled Infliximab Therapy in Patients with Crohn's Disease to Prevent Loss of Response. Dig Dis Sci. 2015 May 23;60(5):1382-8.

[79] Nguyen DL, Palmer LB, Nguyen ET, McClave SA, Martindale RG, Bechtold ML. Specialized enteral nutrition therapy in Crohn's disease patients on maintenance infliximab therapy: a meta-analysis. Therap Adv Gastroenterol. 2015 Jul 25;8(4):168-75.

[80] Sazuka S, Katsuno T, Nakagawa T, Saito M, Saito K, Matsumura T, et al. Concomitant use of enteral nutrition therapy is associated with sustained response to infliximab in patients with Crohn's disease. Eur J Clin Nutr. 2012 Nov 26;66(11):1219-23.

[81] Tanaka T, Takahama K, Kimura T, Mizuno T, Nagasaka M, Iwata K, et al. Effect of concurrent elemental diet on infliximab treatment for Crohn's disease. J Gastroenterol Hepatol. 2006 Jul;21(7):1143-9.

[82] Lemaitre M, Kirchgesner J, Rudnichi A, Carrat F, Zureik M, Carbonnel F, et al. Association Between Use of Thiopurines or Tumor Necrosis Factor Antagonists Alone or in Combination and Risk of Lymphoma in Patients With Inflammatory Bowel Disease. JAMA. 2017 Nov 7;318(17):1679.

[83] Ikeuchi H, Yamamura T, Nakano H, Kosaka T, Shimoyama T, Fukuda Y. Efficacy of nutritional therapy for perforating and non-perforating Crohn's disease. Hepatogastroenterology. 2004;51(58):1050-2.

[84] Esaki M, Matsumoto T, Hizawa K, Nakamura S, Jo Y, Mibu R, et al. Preventive effect of nutritional therapy against postoperative recurrence of Crohn disease, with reference to findings determined by intra-operative enteroscopy. Scand J Gastroenterol. 2005 Jan 8;40(12):1431-7.

[85] Yamamoto T, Nakahigashi M, Umegae S, Kitagawa T, Matsumozo K. Impact of long-term enteral nutrition on clinical and endoscopic recurrence after resection for Crohn's disease: a prospective, non-randomized, parallel, controlled study. Aliment Pharmacol Ther. 2006 Dec 6;25(1):67-72.

[86] Navarro J, Vargas J, Cezard JP, Charritat JL, Polonovski C. Prolonged constant rate elemental enteral

nutrition in Crohn's disease. J Pediatr Gastroenterol Nutr. 1982;1(4):541-6.

[87] Belli DC, Seidman E, Bouthillier L, Weber AM, Roy CC, Pletincx M, et al. Chronic intermittent elemental diet improves growth failure in children with Crohn's disease. Gastroenterology. 1988 Mar;94(3):603-10.

[88] Konno M, Takahashi M, Toita N, Fujiwara S, Nojima M. Long-term therapeutic effectiveness of maintenance enteral nutrition for Crohn's disease. Pediatr Int. 2015 Apr;57(2):276-80.

[89] Schulman JM, Pritzker L, Shaoul R. Maintenance of Remission with Partial Enteral Nutrition Therapy in Pediatric Crohn's Disease: A Retrospective Study. Can J Gastroenterol Hepatol. 2017;2017:1-7.

[90] El-Matary W, Otley A, Critch J, Abou-Setta AM. Enteral Feeding Therapy for Maintaining Remission in Crohn's Disease: A Systematic Review. J Parenter Enter Nutr. 2017 May 8;41(4):550-61.

[91] Gavin J, Marino L V, Ashton JJ, Beattie RM. Patient, parent and professional perception of the use of maintenance enteral nutrition in Paediatric Crohn's Disease. Acta Paediatr. 2018 Dec;107(12):2199-206.

[92] Kim HJ, Kim Y, Cho JM, Oh SH, Kim KM. Therapeutic Efficacy of Oral Enteral Nutrition in Pediatric Crohn's Disease: A Single Center Non-Comparative Retrospective Study. Yonsei Med J [Internet]. 2016 Sep;57(5):1185-91. Available from: https://doi.org/10.3349/ymj.2016.57.5.1185

[93] Watanabe O, Ando T, Ishiguro K, Takahashi H, Ishikawa D, Miyake N, et al. Enteral nutrition decreases hospitalization rate in patients with Crohn's disease. J Gastroenterol Hepatol. 2010 May;25 Suppl 1:S134-7.

Chapter 5

Apheresis in Inflammatory Bowel Disease: Current Evidence

Daniel Vasile Balaban and Mariana Jinga

Abstract

Inflammatory bowel diseases (IBD) have become a major focus for gastroenterologists worldwide, with the increasing incidence and complexity of cases, which pose therapeutic challenges. Currently available approaches fail in controlling the disease activity in a significant proportion of patients and some of the therapies are associated with significant adverse events. Although new molecules are on the horizon and treatment strategies have been optimized, novel therapeutic tools are much needed in IBD for patients who fail to attain control of the disease. Apheresis is now a common non-pharmacological therapeutic modality used in several pathologies, IBD also. In the current review, we summarize currently available evidence with respect to selective apheresis in IBD.

Keywords: inflammatory bowel disease, ulcerative colitis, Crohn's disease, apheresis, leukapheresis

1. Introduction

Inflammatory bowel diseases (IBD), comprising ulcerative colitis (UC) and Crohn's disease (CD), are chronic inflammatory conditions of the digestive tract with a relapsing-remitting course, which can dramatically decrease patients' quality of life. With a steadily increasing incidence worldwide [1] and with the growing needs and demands from patients, IBD have become a major focus for the gastroenterology community, both practitioners and researchers. Over the last decades, management of IBD has improved considerably, but is quite far from being satisfactory for a significant number of patients. Currently, the therapeutic armamentarium includes several drug regimens, endoscopic therapies, and surgery. Despite the development of novel targeted molecules and optimization of treatment strategies in IBD, some patients fail to achieve disease control with currently available treatment options. Moreover, drug-based therapies are associated with significant adverse events and contraindications, which may lead to treatment discontinuation or even refusal of therapy. Not least, chronic use of conventional therapies is associated with loss of response, which can pose challenges in the long-term control of the disease. In this setting, novel therapeutic approaches have been searched for by the scientific community and apheresis has emerged as a promising non-pharmacologic treatment option in IBD.

Although guidelines are not frequently reporting it [2], several successful experiences have been reported so far in the literature. In this chapter, we will summarize current evidence regarding apheresis in IBD.

2. Principles of apheresis in IBD

Apheresis techniques are being used in many medical specialties, from nephrology and intensive care to gastroenterology. It consists of depleting the patient's blood from certain components (cells, cytokines, or other molecules) depending of the filter used and the indication. Its applications in digestive pathology include alcoholic hepatitis [3], hepatitis C-associated cryoglobulinemia [4], hypertriglyceridemia-induced acute pancreatitis [5], and IBD.

IBD is undoubtedly characterized by complex pathogenesis, but leucocytes play a key role in driving the bowel inflammation. Most of the conventional treatments in IBD address the proinflammatory cytokines released by the activated leucocytes, while apheresis acts by extracting the white cells (specifically a subset of WBCs) from the patient's blood, either by centrifugation or by passing the blood through an adsorptive device. Initially, centrifugation was used to deplete the activated leukocytes from the patient's blood; this reduction in the number of WBCs proved beneficial for IBD patients but had limitations generated from the nonspecific removal of leukocytes. To overcome these limitations, columns containing membrane filters or adsorbing beads have been developed to selectively remove the desired level of WBCs.

Regarding the use of apheresis in IBD, its benefits reside from depleting the blood from certain subtypes of leucocytes, which migrate into the bowel wall and fuel the local inflammatory response. This selective removal of specific white cells—mostly granulocytes and monocytes—is being regarded as a technique of extracorporeal immunomodulation, with proven benefits for IBD patients; besides this selective depletion of granulocytes and monocytes/macrophages, several other beneficial changes in the inflammatory cascade of IBD patients have been reported and could contribute to the efficacy of apheresis in IBD [6].

A schematic description of leukocyte apheresis in IBD is represented in **Figure 1**—the patients' blood is passed through a filter which selectively removes white cells (mainly granulocytes and monocytes) and then returned to the patient's body; the resulting blood has fewer leukocytes and in turn there are (?) less of them to fuel the inflammation in the bowel wall. As for other extracorporeal machines, anticoagulation is used during leukapheresis for IBD.

First reports of apheresis in IBD date back from 1980s [7], when centrifugal leukocytapheresis was used in patients with Crohn's disease. With this technique, the patient's blood was depleted by about 55% of lymphocytes, 40% of granulocytes, and a significant amount of red blood cells and platelets [6].

Subsequent models for apheresis incorporated a filter or a column for the selective removal of certain blood components. Currently, there are two leukocyte adsorptive devices available for apheresis in IBD patients [6, 8]:

- *Adacolumn* (Japan Immunoresearch Laboratory, Japan), a granulocyte/monocyte apheresis (GMA) system which consists of a column filled with cellulose-coated acetate beads that selectively remove granulocytes and monocytes through binding of FCγR (Fc gamma receptor—a receptor for the Fc portion of IgG), and to a lesser extent lymphocytes, as they do not express FCγR [9]. The device adsorbs 65% of granulocytes, 55% of monocytes, and only 2% of lymphocytes and few platelets [10]. Patients usually undergo one or more sessions per week up, according to different protocols.

- *Cellsorba* (Asahi Medical, Japan), a leukocyte apheresis (LCAP) system represented by a column containing non-woven polyester fibers, which retain leucocytes as follows: 90–100% of granulocytes and monocytes, 30–60% of lymphocytes, and a certain amount of thrombocytes [11, 12].

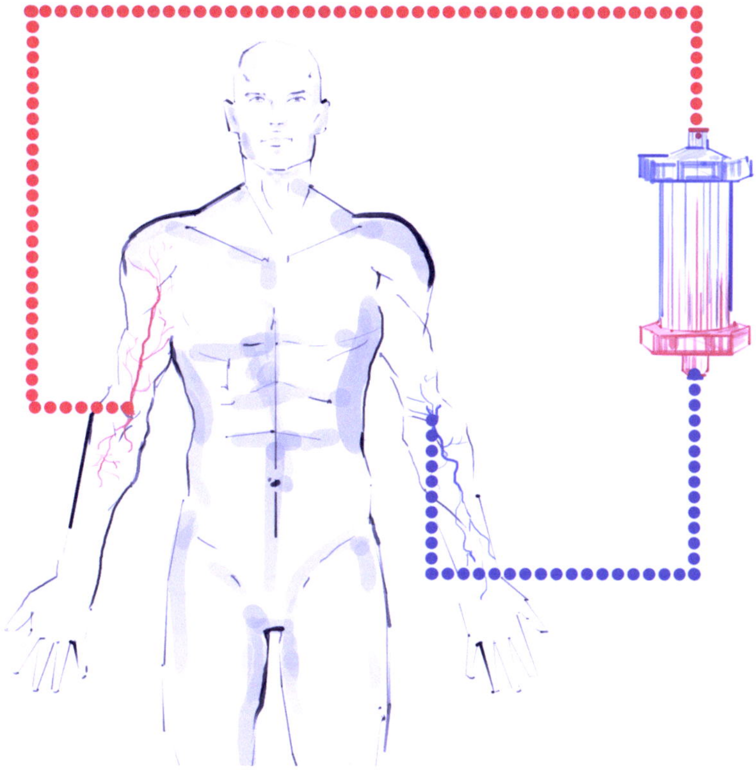

Figure 1.
Schematic representation of apheresis in IBD.

3. Leukapheresis in IBD

Leukocyte apheresis (leukapheresis) has been evaluated in several trials as a treatment option in patients with steroid-dependent or steroid-refractory UC/CD and in moderate-severe disease unresponsive to conventional therapy. The standard protocol implies that the patient has one apheresis session (60 minutes duration) per week for 5–10 consecutive weeks, but others have proposed modified protocols with more intensive therapy (2 sessions per week, 90 minutes duration). Common adverse reactions include dizziness, headache, and mild, transient fever. The procedure has a good safety profile and is usually well tolerated. Leukapheresis allows IBD patients to taper or even get off steroids and to achieve earlier remission [13]. Besides patients with steroid-dependent and steroid-refractory disease, it has proven efficacious in steroid-native patients also. A major issue of leukapheresis is cost, but considering the elimination of the need for steroids and their complications and the need for hospitalization for flaring, this non-pharmacologic technique may be cost-effective for selected patient categories [14]. A selection of studies reporting its efficacy and safety is presented in **Tables 1** and **2**.

Most of the above papers report on the efficacy and safety of apheresis techniques in difficult to treat patient categories—steroid-dependent/-resistant or refractory to conventional treatment, UC being studied more than CD. However, while early observational studies have reported very high response or remission rates (up to 80%) in these difficult to treat patients, a randomized controlled trial comparing GMA to sham (placebo) showed much lower remission rates and no significant differences between the compared groups than in previous studies [36].

Author, year	Indication	No. of patients	Overall response rate	Adverse events (number or %)
Shimoyama et al., 2001 [15]	UC (refractory to conventional treatment)	53	58.5% of patients had remission or improved	9.4%—8 non-severe AE (in 5 patients)
Tomomasa et al., 2003 [16]	Pediatric UC (steroid-refractory)	12	67% improvement	9%
Hanai et al., 2003 [17]	UC	31 steroid-refractory 8 steroid naive	81% remission in steroid-refractory, 88% in steroid-naive	18%
Matsui et al., 2003 [18]	CD (refractory to conventional treatment)	7	71.4%	
Hanai et al., 2004 [19]	UC (steroid-dependent)	46	83% remission at week 12	21.7% (10 mild AE)
Suzuki et al., 2004 [20]	UC (steroid-naive)	20	85% remission	10%
Kusaka et al., 2004 [21]	CD (un-responsive to conventional treatment)	6	66.6%	
Fukuda et al., 2004 [22]	CD (moderate-severe, unresponsive to standard therapy)	21	52.4%	
Naganuma et al., 2004 [23]	UC (steroid-refractory or -dependent)	44	55% remission + 20% clinical response	5%
Yamamoto et al., 2004 [24]	UC (mild-moderate)	30	70% clinical remission	27% (in 8 patients, 9 sessions)
Domenench 2004 [25]	UC and CD	14 (13*) UC, 12 (10*) CD	62% remission in UC, 70% in CD	4
Kanke et al., 2004 [26]	UC (mild to severe)	60	23% remission, 60% improvement	18%
Kim et al., 2005 [27]	UC (refractory to conventional treatment)	27	70% improvement	11%
Kruis et al., 2005 [28]	UC	39 (35*)	37.1% clinical remission and 28.6% endoscopic remission	1
D'Ovidio et al., 2006 [29]	UC (mild-moderate, steroid dependent/ refractory)	12	75% clinical response	None
Ikeda et al., 2006 [30]	Pediatric UC	4	75%	
Sands et al., 2006 [31]	IBD	15 UC, 15 CD	Response—45.5% UC, 64.3% CD	No SAE
Muratov et al., 2006 [32]	IBD (relapse or refractory to conventional treatment)	10 (7 CD, 3 UC)	50% remission	No SAE

Author, year	Indication	No. of patients	Overall response rate	Adverse events (number or %)
Ljung et al., 2007 [33]	UC, CD, and indeterminate colitis (mostly steroid-refractory or steroid-dependent)	100	69% remission or response	15
Yamamoto et al., 2007 [34]	UC	50	52% clinical remission, 34% endoscopic remission	
Bresci et al., 2007 [35]	UC	40	70% clinical response	1
Sands et al., 2008 [36]	UC (moderate-severe)	169	17% clinical remission in GMA-group (vs 11% sham-treatment group)	—
Maiden et al., 2008 [37]	UC and CD	29	72.4% clinical remission at 6 months	55% mild and transient headache No SAE
Hanai et al., 2008 [38]	UC (moderate or severe)	70 (35 randomized to Adacolumn)	74.3% clinical remission at 12 weeks	5 mild AE 2 discontinued
Tanaka et al., 2008 [39]	UC	45	73.3% clinical remission	No SAE Transient flushing and light-headedness in few patients
Sakata et al., 2008 [40]	UC (moderate-severe)	39 randomized (17 Adacolumn, 21 Cellsorba)	76.5% clinical improvement in Adacolumn-group, 66.7% in Cellsorba-group	No SAE
de Carpi et al., 2008 [41]	Pediatric IBD	9 (5 UC, 4 CD)	55.5% remission	No SAE
Hibi et al., 2009 [42]	UC (severe, refractory to conventional medications)	697	77.3%	7.7% mild-moderate No SAE
Sakuraba et al., 2009 [43]	UC (mild-to-moderately active UC)	163	Clinical remission—54.0% in weekly GMA and 71.2% in intensive GMA	No GMA-related SAE
Cabriada et al., 2010 [44]	UC (steroid-dependent)	18 (Cellsorba—2, Adacolumn—16)	55% clinical remission (induction), 50% endoscopic remission	None
Yamamoto et al., 2010 [45]	UC (endoscopically active)	124	45% clinical remission	

Author, year	Indication	No. of patients	Overall response rate	Adverse events (number or %)
Lindberg et al., 2010 [46]	IBD (unresponsive to conventional treatment)	15 UC, 25 CD	85% clinical response, 65% complete remission	6 AE No SAE
Bresci et al., 2010 [47]	Refractory CD	16	63.3% clinical remission	No SAE
D'Ovidio et al., 2011 [48]	UC (steroid dependent/refractory)	69	58% responders	2 mild, 1 transient arrhythmia
Cabriada et al., 2012 [49]	UC (steroid-dependent)	142	41% remission at 6 months, 36% remission at 12 months	1 SAE
Yokoyama et al., 2013 [50]	UC	43	53.5% clinical remission rate	No SAE
Sacco et al., 2013 [51]	IBD	118 (83 UC, 35 CD)	71% UC clinical remission, 63% CD	
Fukuchi et al., 2014 [52]	CD	22	81.8% clinical remission at 52 weeks	No SAE
Yoshimura et al., 2015 [53]	CD (moderate-severe)	104	Remission—35.6% in weekly GMA, 35.2% in intensive GMA	22.2%
Tanida et al., 2015 [54]	Refractory UC	9	55.6% cumulative clinical remission at 10 weeks	3
Kruis et al., 2015 [55]	UC	168 (165*—68 with microscopic erosion/ ulceration)	23.9% remission with GMA vs. 0% sham	
Dignass et al., 2016 [56]	UC (steroid-dependent, moderate-to-severe, with insufficient response or intolerance to immunosuppressants and/or biologics)	86	39.3% clinical remission, 56% clinical response	Majority mild-moderate
Ruuska et al., 2016 [57]	Pediatric UC	25	45% significant improvement, 25% moderate improvement	21 AE in 8/25 (32%), no SAE
Imperiali et al., 2017 [58]	UC (moderate, steroid-dependent, azathioprine-intolerant/ resistant)	33	36% steroid-free clinical remission at 1 year +9% clinical response	1
Lai et al., 2017 [59]	UC	34	70.59% overall efficacy	No GMA-related SAE

Author, year	Indication	No. of patients	Overall response rate	Adverse events (number or %)
Motoya et al., 2019 [60]	UC and CD	437	46.4% clinical remission in UC, 33.3% in CD	11.4%

Overall response rate—response + remission rate.
GMA—granulocyte and monocyte/macrophage apheresis, AE—adverse events, SAE— severe adverse events, UC—ulcerative colitis.
**Number of patients included in the final analysis.*

Table 1.
Summary of studies reporting the efficacy of Adacolumn in IBD.

Author, year	Indication	No of patients	Overall response rate	Adverse events (number or %)
Kosaka et al., 1999 [61]	CD (refractory to conventional treatment)	18	50%	
Sawada et al., 1995 [62]	Both UC and CD	44 (25 UC, 19 CD)	Clinical improvement—85% in UC, 84.2% in CD	
Sawada et al., 2003 [63]	UC	39	74%	28%
Sawada et al., 2005 [64]	UC (moderate-to-severe)	25 (9 excluded; 10 randomized to active-group, 9 sham)	80% clinical improvement	1
Sawada et al., 2005 [65]	UC with toxic megacolon	6	66.7% improved, 33.3% colectomy	
Nishioka et al., 2005 [66]	UC	29 (9 LCAP, 20 cortisone)	88.9% clinical improvement, 35% remission	No major AE
Takemoto et al., 2007 [67]	UC (steroid-resistant)	71	75% initial response, 27% maintained remission >6 months	4%
Emmrich et al., 2007 [68]	UC (refractory to conventional treatment)	20	70% clinical remission	
Shimada et al., 2008 [69]	UC (moderate-to-severe)	10	80% clinical remission	None
Yokoyama et al., 2014 [70]	UC	847 (623*)	68.9% overall clinical remission, 62.5% mucosal healing	10.3% of which 0.6% severe
Kobayashi et al., 2018 [71]	UC	314	63.6% 1-year cumulative relapse-free rate, 85.1% response rate in re-treatment	

Overall response rate—response + remission rate.
AE—adverse events, SAE—severe adverse events.
**Number of patients included in the final analysis.*

Table 2.
Summary of studies reporting the efficacy of Cellsorba in IBD.

Along with the observational nature of most studies on apheresis in IBD, another important limit is that many of them were conducted in the era before biologics and novel oral therapies for IBD, when patients did not have so many options when failing steroids. While early studies evaluated the efficacy of apheresis as monotherapy in refractory IBD, more recent ones have proposed combination therapy of biologics with adsorptive apheresis, with promising results [72]. Also, recent studies have shown good results not only in induction of remission but also as maintenance therapy [73].

Not least, another limitation is that a significant proportion of studies report on small sample sizes, with very heterogeneous study groups with regard to severity and extent of disease, which limit on extrapolation of the results in all patient categories. There are some studies on special patient populations such as the elderly and pediatric/adolescent patients, in whom adverse reactions of conventional therapy can be more severe or even contraindicate their use [60].

With regard to safety, most of the adverse effects reported were mild and transient (such as fever, headache, flushing, and dizziness), very rarely severe adverse events. Despite being an invasive procedure, a study looking at the patients' perspective found that GMA is well accepted by patients suffering from IBD [74]. This is very encouraging considering that up to one in two patients encounter side effects with conventional therapies [15].

Regarding the type of anticoagulant used for the extracorporeal circulation of the blood during the apheresis session, there is one comparative study looking at nafamostat mesilate versus heparin, the latter being associated with a lower rate of AE [75].

In order to improve the outcome and safety of the procedure, some authors have also looked at the optimal apheresis treatment volume, showing that using a bodyweight adjusted volume is associated with similar therapeutic efficacy but with less AE [76].

Considering the current evidence, with the wide range of results from very heterogeneous studies, the upcoming research should focus on establishing markers to appropriately select IBD patients that would safely and cost-effective benefit from apheresis techniques [77].

Besides GMA and LCAP, novel apheresis techniques are being studied in IBD such as leucocyte/thrombocyte apheresis system, which showed promising results in a small prospective, randomized, controlled multicenter pilot study [78].

4. Conclusions

While leukocyte-derived proinflammatory cytokines have been validated as successful targets in IBD treatment, so should leukocytes themselves be considered as treatment options. As activated leukocytes migrate into the bowel wall and drive the inflammatory cascade in IBD patients, their depletion by apheresis techniques are considered beneficial to control the mucosal inflammation.

Leukapheresis, consisting in either granulomonocyte apheresis or leukocyte apheresis, are cell-based therapies with promising results in some patient categories and with a good safety profile. They have been studied as an alternative in patients with steroid toxicity, dependency or refractoriness, or in the event of contraindications to conventional therapy. Most of the early studies were not controlled, with only a few randomized controlled trials providing quality data on their efficacy. Future studies should be designed to look at selection of IBD patients who benefit most and safely from this non-pharmacological therapy.

Author details

Daniel Vasile Balaban[1,2*] and Mariana Jinga[1,2]

1 "Carol Davila" University of Medicine and Pharmacy, Bucharest, Romania

2 "Dr. Carol Davila" Central Military Emergency University Hospital, Bucharest, Romania

*Address all correspondence to: vbalaban@yahoo.com

References

[1] GBD 2017 Inflammatory Bowel Disease Collaborators. The global, regional, and national burden of inflammatory bowel disease in 195 countries and territories, 1990-2017: A systematic analysis for the Global Burden of Disease Study 2017. The Lancet Gastroenterology & Hepatology. 2020;**5**(1):17-30. DOI: 10.1016/S2468-1253(19)30333-4

[2] Torres J, Bonovas S, Doherty G, et al. ECCO guidelines on therapeutics in Crohn's disease: Medical treatment. Journal of Crohn's & Colitis. 2020;**14**(1):4-22. DOI: 10.1093/ecco-jcc/jjz180

[3] Parés A, Mas A. Extracorporeal liver support in severe alcoholic hepatitis. World Journal of Gastroenterology. 2014;**20**(25):8011-8017. DOI: 10.3748/wjg.v20.i25.8011

[4] Montero N, Favà A, Rodriguez E, et al. Treatment for hepatitis C virus-associated mixed cryoglobulinaemia. Cochrane Database of Systematic Reviews. 2018;**5**(5):CD011403. DOI: 10.1002/14651858.CD011403.pub2

[5] Joglekar K, Brannick B, Kadaria D, Sodhi A. Therapeutic plasmapheresis for hypertriglyceridemia-associated acute pancreatitis: Case series and review of the literature. Therapeutic Advances in Endocrinology and Metabolism. 2017;**8**(4):59-65. DOI: 10.1177/2042018817695449

[6] Danese S, Angelucci E, Stefanelli T, et al. Cytapheresis in inflammatory bowel diseases: Current evidence and perspectives. Digestion. 2008;**77**(2):96-107. DOI: 10.1159/000122473

[7] Bicks RO, Groshart KD. The current status of T-lymphocyte apheresis (TLA) treatment of Crohn's disease. Journal of Clinical Gastroenterology. 1989;**11**(2):136-138

[8] Staley EM et al. Therapeutic leukocyte apheresis and absorptive cytapheresis. In: Transfusion Medicine and Hemostatis. 3rd ed. Elsevier; 2019

[9] Saniabadi AR, Hanai H, Takeuchi K, et al. Adacolumn, an adsorptive carrier based granulocyte and monocyte apheresis device for the treatment of inflammatory and refractory diseases associated with leukocytes. Therapeutic Apheresis and Dialysis. 2003;**7**:48-59

[10] Hibi T, Sakuraba A. Is there a role for apheresis in gastrointestinal disorders? Nature Clinical Practice. Gastroenterology & Hepatology. 2005;**2**(5):200-201. DOI: 10.1038/ncpgasthep0168

[11] Shirokaze J. Leukocytapheresis using a leukocyte removal filter. Therapeutic Apheresis. 2002;**6**:261-266

[12] Shibata H, Kuriyama T, Yamawaki N. Cellsorba. Therapeutic Apheresis and Dialysis. 2003;**7**:44-47

[13] Iizuka M, Etou T, Kumagai M, Matsuoka A, Numata Y, Sagara S. Long-interval cytapheresis as a novel therapeutic strategy leading to dosage reduction and discontinuation of steroids in steroid-dependent ulcerative colitis. Internal Medicine. 2017;**56**(20):2705-2710. DOI: 10.2169/internalmedicine.8428-16

[14] Yamamoto T, Umegae S, Matsumoto K. Safety and clinical efficacy of granulocyte and monocyte adsorptive apheresis therapy for ulcerative colitis. World Journal of Gastroenterology. 2006;**12**(4):520-525. DOI: 10.3748/wjg.v12.i4.520

[15] Shimoyama T, Sawada K, Hiwatashi N, et al. Safety and efficacy of granulocyte and monocyte adsorption apheresis in patients with active ulcerative colitis: A multicenter

study. Journal of Clinical Apheresis. 2001;**16**(1):1-9. DOI: 10.1002/jca.1000

[16] Tomomasa T, Kobayashi A, Kaneko H, et al. Granulocyte adsorptive apheresis for pediatric patients with ulcerative colitis. Digestive Diseases and Sciences. 2003;**48**(4):750-754. DOI: 10.1023/a:1022892927121

[17] Hanai H, Watanabe F, Takeuchi K, Iida T, Yamada M, Iwaoka Y, et al. Leukocyte adsorptive apheresis for the treatment of active ulcerative colitis: A prospective, uncontrolled, pilot study. Clinical Gastroenterology and Hepatology. 2003;**1**:28-35

[18] Matsui T, Nishimura T, Matake H, Ohta T, Sakurai T, Yao T. Granulocytapheresis for Crohn's disease: A report on seven refractory patients. The American Journal of Gastroenterology. 2003;**98**(2):511-512. DOI: 10.1111/j.1572-0241.2003.07251.x

[19] Hanai H, Watanabe F, Yamada M, et al. Adsorptive granulocyte and monocyte apheresis versus prednisolone in patients with corticosteroid-dependent moderately severe ulcerative colitis. Digestion. 2004;**70**(1):36-44. DOI: 10.1159/000080079

[20] Suzuki Y, Yoshimura N, Saniabadi AR, Saito Y. Selective granulocyte and monocyte adsorptive apheresis as a first-line treatment for steroid naïve patients with active ulcerative colitis: A prospective uncontrolled study. Digestive Diseases and Sciences. 2004;**49**:565-571

[21] Kusaka T, Fukunaga K, Ohnishi K, et al. Adsorptive monocyte-granulocytapheresis (M-GCAP) for refractory Crohn's disease. Journal of Clinical Apheresis. 2004;**19**(4):168-173. DOI: 10.1002/jca.20023

[22] Fukuda Y, Matsui T, Suzuki Y, et al. Adsorptive granulocyte and monocyte apheresis for refractory Crohn's disease: An open multicenter prospective study. Journal of Gastroenterology. 2004;**39**(12):1158-1164. DOI: 10.1007/s00535-004-1465-z

[23] Naganuma M, Funakoshi S, Sakuraba A, Takagi H, Inoue N, Ogata H, et al. Granulocytapheresis is useful as an alternative therapy in patients with steroid-refractory or -dependent ulcerative colitis. Inflammatory Bowel Diseases. 2004;**10**:251-257

[24] Yamamoto T, Umegae S, Kitagawa T, Yasuda Y, Yamada Y, Takahashi D, et al. Granulocyte and monocyte adsorptive apheresis in the treatment of active distal ulcerative colitis: A prospective, pilot study. Alimentary Pharmacology & Therapeutics. 2004;**20**:783-792

[25] Domènech E, Hinojosa J, Esteve-Comas M, et al. Granulocyteaphaeresis in steroid-dependent inflammatory bowel disease: A prospective, open, pilot study. Alimentary Pharmacology & Therapeutics. 2004;**20**(11-12):1347-1352. DOI: 10.1111/j.1365-2036.2004.02288.x

[26] Kanke K, Nakano M, Hiraishi H, Terano A. Clinical evaluation of granulocyte/monocyte apheresis therapy for active ulcerative colitis. Digestive and Liver Disease. 2004;**36**:811-817

[27] Kim HJ, Kim JS, Han DS, Yang SK, Hahm KB, Lee WI, et al. Granulocyte and monocyte adsorption apheresis in Korean conventional treatment-refractory patients with active ulcerative colitis: A prospective open-label multicenter study. The Korean Journal of Gastroenterology. 2005;**45**:34-44

[28] Kruis W, Dignass A, Steinhagen-Thiessen E, et al. Open label trial of granulocyte apheresis suggests therapeutic efficacy in chronically active steroid refractory ulcerative colitis. World Journal of Gastroenterology.

2005;**11**(44):7001-7006. DOI: 10.3748/wjg.v11.i44.7001

[29] D'Ovidio V, Aratari A, Viscido A, et al. Mucosal features and granulocyte-monocyte-apheresis in steroid-dependent/refractory ulcerative colitis. Digestive and Liver Disease. 2006;**38**(6):389-394. DOI: 10.1016/j.dld.2005.12.005

[30] Ikeda H, Ishimaru Y, Takayasu H, et al. Efficacy of granulocyte apheresis in pediatric patients with ulcerative colitis: A pilot study. Journal of Pediatric Gastroenterology and Nutrition. 2006;**43**(5):592-596. DOI: 10.1097/01.mpg.0000237928.07729.79

[31] Sands BE, Sandborn WJ, Wolf DC, et al. Pilot feasibility studies of leukocytapheresis with the Adacolumn apheresis system in patients with active ulcerative colitis or Crohn disease. Journal of Clinical Gastroenterology. 2006;**40**(6):482-489. DOI: 10.1097/00004836-200607000-00005

[32] Muratov V, Lundahl J, Ulfgren AK, et al. Down-regulation of interferon-gamma parallels clinical response to selective leukocyte apheresis in patients with inflammatory bowel disease: A 12-month follow-up study. International Journal of Colorectal Disease. 2006;**21**(6):493-504. DOI: 10.1007/s00384-005-0069-2

[33] Ljung T, Thomsen OØ, Vatn M, et al. Granulocyte, monocyte/macrophage apheresis for inflammatory bowel disease: The first 100 patients treated in Scandinavia. Scandinavian Journal of Gastroenterology. 2007;**42**(2):221-227. DOI: 10.1080/00365520600979369

[34] Yamamoto T, Saniabadi AR, Maruyama Y, Umegae S, Matsumoto K. Factors affecting clinical and endoscopic efficacies of selective leucocytapheresis for ulcerative colitis. Digestive and Liver Disease. 2007;**39**(7):626-633. DOI: 10.1016/j.dld.2007.04.007

[35] Bresci G, Parisi G, Mazzoni A, Scatena F, Capria A. Treatment of patients with acute ulcerative colitis: Conventional corticosteroid therapy (MP) versus granulocytapheresis (GMA): A pilot study. Digestive and Liver Disease. 2007;**39**(5):430-434. DOI: 10.1016/j.dld.2007.01.001

[36] Sands BE, Sandborn WJ, Feagan B, et al. A randomized, double-blind, sham-controlled study of granulocyte/monocyte apheresis for active ulcerative colitis. Gastroenterology. 2008;**135**(2):400-409. DOI: 10.1053/j.gastro.2008.04.023

[37] Maiden L, Takeuchi K, Baur R, et al. Selective white cell apheresis reduces relapse rates in patients with IBD at significant risk of clinical relapse. Inflammatory Bowel Diseases. 2008;**14**(10):1413-1418. DOI: 10.1002/ibd.20505

[38] Hanai H, Iida T, Takeuchi K, et al. Intensive granulocyte and monocyte adsorption versus intravenous prednisolone in patients with severe ulcerative colitis: An unblinded randomised multi-centre controlled study. Digestive and Liver Disease. 2008;**40**(6):433-440. DOI: 10.1016/j.dld.2008.01.007

[39] Tanaka T, Okanobu H, Yoshimi S, et al. In patients with ulcerative colitis, adsorptive depletion of granulocytes and monocytes impacts mucosal level of neutrophils and clinically is most effective in steroid naïve patients. Digestive and Liver Disease. 2008;**40**(9):731-736. DOI: 10.1016/j.dld.2008.02.012

[40] Sakata Y, Iwakiri R, Amemori S, et al. Comparison of the efficacy of granulocyte and monocyte/macrophage adsorptive apheresis and leukocytapheresis in active ulcerative colitis patients: A prospective randomized study. European Journal of Gastroenterology & Hepatology.

2008;**20**(7):629-633. DOI: 10.1097/MEG.0b013e3282f5e9a4

[41] Martín de Carpi J, Vilar P, Prieto G, García Novo MD, Ribes C, Varea V. Safety and efficacy of granulocyte and monocyte adsorption apheresis in paediatric inflammatory bowel disease: A prospective pilot study. Journal of Pediatric Gastroenterology and Nutrition. 2008;**46**(4):386-391. DOI: 10.1097/MPG.0b013e31815604e5

[42] Hibi T, Sameshima Y, Sekiguchi Y, et al. Treating ulcerative colitis by Adacolumn therapeutic leucocytapheresis: Clinical efficacy and safety based on surveillance of 656 patients in 53 centres in Japan. Digestive and Liver Disease. 2009;**41**(8):570-577. DOI: 10.1016/j.dld.2008.11.020

[43] Sakuraba A, Motoya S, Watanabe K, et al. An open-label prospective randomized multicenter study shows very rapid remission of ulcerative colitis by intensive granulocyte and monocyte adsorptive apheresis as compared with routine weekly treatment. The American Journal of Gastroenterology. 2009;**104**(12):2990-2995. DOI: 10.1038/ajg.2009.453

[44] Cabriada JL, Ibargoyen N, Hernández A, Bernal A, Castiella A. Sustained remission after steroids and leukocytapheresis induced response in steroid-dependent ulcerative colitis: Results at 1 year. Digestive and Liver Disease. 2010;**42**(6):432-435. DOI: 10.1016/j.dld.2009.09.001

[45] Yamamoto T, Umegae S, Matsumoto K. Mucosal healing in patients with ulcerative colitis during a course of selective leukocytapheresis therapy: A prospective cohort study. Inflammatory Bowel Diseases. 2010;**16**(11):1905-1911. DOI: 10.1002/ibd.21260

[46] Lindberg A, Eberhardson M, Karlsson M, Karlén P. Long-term follow-up with granulocyte and monocyte apheresis re-treatment in patients with chronically active inflammatory bowel disease. BMC Gastroenterology. 2010;**10**:73. DOI: 10.1186/1471-230X-10-73

[47] Bresci G, Romano A, Mazzoni A, et al. Feasibility and safety of granulocytapheresis in Crohn's disease: A prospective cohort study. Gastroentérologie Clinique et Biologique. 2010;**34**(12):682-686. DOI: 10.1016/j.gcb.2010.09.009

[48] D'Ovidio V, Meo D, Viscido A, Bresci G, Vernia P, Caprilli R. Predictive factors of clinical response in steroid-refractory ulcerative colitis treated with granulocyte-monocyte apheresis. World Journal of Gastroenterology. 2011;**17**(14):1831-1835. DOI: 10.3748/wjg.v17.i14.1831

[49] Cabriada JL, Domènech E, Ibargoyen N, et al. Leukocytapheresis for steroid-dependent ulcerative colitis in clinical practice: Results of a nationwide Spanish registry. Journal of Gastroenterology. 2012;**47**(4):359-365. DOI: 10.1007/s00535-011-0499-2

[50] Yokoyama Y, Kawai M, Fukunaga K, et al. Looking for predictive factors of clinical response to adsorptive granulocyte and monocyte apheresis in patients with ulcerative colitis: markers of response to GMA. BMC Gastroenterology. 2013;**13**:27. DOI: 10.1186/1471-230X-13-27

[51] Sacco R, Romano A, Mazzoni A, et al. Granulocytapheresis in steroid-dependent and steroid-resistant patients with inflammatory bowel disease: A prospective observational study. Journal of Crohn's & Colitis. 2013;**7**(12):e692-e697. DOI: 10.1016/j.crohns.2013.06.012

[52] Fukuchi T, Nakase H, Ubukata S, et al. Therapeutic effect of intensive granulocyte and monocyte adsorption

apheresis combined with thiopurines for steroid- and biologics-naïve Japanese patients with early-diagnosed Crohn's disease. BMC Gastroenterology. 2014;**13**:124. DOI: 10.1186/1471-230X-14-124

[53] Yoshimura N, Yokoyama Y, Matsuoka K, et al. An open-label prospective randomized multicenter study of intensive versus weekly granulocyte and monocyte apheresis in active Crohn's disease. BMC Gastroenterology. 2015;**15**:163. DOI: 10.1186/s12876-015-0390-3

[54] Tanida S, Mizoshita T, Nishie H, et al. Combination therapy with adalimumab plus intensive granulocyte and monocyte adsorptive apheresis in patients with refractory ulcerative colitis. Journal of Clinical Medical Research. 2015;**7**(11):884-889. DOI: 10.14740/jocmr2333w

[55] Kruis W, Nguyen P, Morgenstern J. Granulocyte/monocyte adsorptive apheresis in moderate to severe ulcerative colitis--Effective or not? Digestion. 2015;**92**(1):39-44. DOI: 10.1159/000431149

[56] Dignass A, Akbar A, Hart A, et al. Safety and efficacy of granulocyte/monocyte apheresis in steroid-dependent active ulcerative colitis with insufficient response or intolerance to immunosuppressants and/or biologics [the ART trial]: 12-week interim results. Journal of Crohn's & Colitis. 2016;**10**(7):812-820. DOI: 10.1093/ecco-jcc/jjw032

[57] Ruuska T, Küster P, Grahnquist L, Lindgren F, Wewer AV. Efficacy and safety of granulocyte, monocyte/macrophage adsorptive in pediatric ulcerative colitis. World Journal of Gastroenterology. 2016;**22**(17):4389-4396. DOI: 10.3748/wjg.v22.i17.4389

[58] Imperiali G, Amato A, Terpin MM, et al. Granulocyte-monocyte apheresis in steroid-dependent, azathioprine-intolerant/resistant moderate ulcerative colitis: A prospective multicenter study. Gastroenterology Research and Practice. 2017;**2017**:9728324. DOI: 10.1155/2017/9728324

[59] Lai YM, Yao WY, He Y, et al. Adsorptive granulocyte and monocyte apheresis in the treatment of ulcerative colitis: The first multicenter study in China. Gut Liver. 2017;**11**(2):216-225. DOI: 10.5009/gnl15408

[60] Motoya S, Tanaka H, Shibuya T, et al. Safety and effectiveness of granulocyte and monocyte adsorptive apheresis in patients with inflammatory bowel disease in special situations: A multicentre cohort study. BMC Gastroenterology. 2019;**19**(1):196. DOI: 10.1186/s12876-019-1110-1

[61] Kosaka T, Sawada K, Ohnishi K, et al. Effect of leukocytapheresis therapy using a leukocyte removal filter in Crohn's disease. Internal Medicine. 1999;**38**(2):102-111. DOI: 10.2169/internalmedicine.38.102

[62] Sawada K, Ohnishi K, Kosaka T, et al. Leukocytapheresis therapy with leukocyte removal filter for inflammatory bowel disease. Journal of Gastroenterology. 1995;**30**(Suppl 8):124-127

[63] Sawada K, Muto T, Shimoyama T, et al. Multicenter randomized controlled trial for the treatment of ulcerative colitis with a leukocytapheresis column. Current Pharmaceutical Design. 2003;**9**(4):307-321. DOI: 10.2174/1381612033391928

[64] Sawada K, Kusugami K, Suzuki Y, et al. Leukocytapheresis in ulcerative colitis: Results of a multicenter double-blind prospective case-control study with sham apheresis as placebo treatment. The American

Journal of Gastroenterology. 2005;**100**(6):1362-1369. DOI: 10.1111/j.1572-0241.2005.41089.x

[65] Sawada K, Egashira A, Ohnishi K, Fukunaga K, Kusaka T, Shimoyama T. Leukocytapheresis (LCAP) for management of fulminant ulcerative colitis with toxic megacolon. Digestive Diseases and Sciences. 2005;**50**(4):767-773. DOI: 10.1007/s10620-005-2571-3

[66] Nishioka C, Aoyama N, Maekawa S, et al. Leukocytapheresis therapy for steroid-naïve patients with active ulcerative colitis: Its clinical efficacy and adverse effects compared with those of conventional steroid therapy. Journal of Gastroenterology and Hepatology. 2005;**20**(10):1567-1571. DOI: 10.1111/j.1440-1746.2005.03907.x

[67] Takemoto K, Kato J, Kuriyama M, et al. Predictive factors of efficacy of leukocytapheresis for steroid-resistant ulcerative colitis patients. Digestive and Liver Disease. 2007;**39**(5):422-429. DOI: 10.1016/j.dld.2007.01.010

[68] Emmrich J, Petermann S, Nowak D, et al. Leukocytapheresis (LCAP) in the management of chronic active ulcerative colitis--Results of a randomized pilot trial. Digestive Diseases and Sciences. 2007;**52**(9):2044-2053. DOI: 10.1007/s10620-006-9696-x

[69] Shimada M, Iwase H, Tsuzuki T, et al. A pilot study of leukocytapheresis efficacy with 1.5 liter blood processing volume in patients with ulcerative colitis. Therapeutic Apheresis and Dialysis. 2008;**12**(5):368-373. DOI: 10.1111/j.1744-9987.2008.00611.x

[70] Yokoyama Y, Matsuoka K, Kobayashi T, et al. A large-scale, prospective, observational study of leukocytapheresis for ulcerative colitis: Treatment outcomes of 847 patients in clinical practice. Journal of Crohn's & Colitis. 2014;**8**(9):981-991. DOI: 10.1016/j.crohns.2014.01.027

[71] Kobayashi T, Matsuoka K, Yokoyama Y, et al. A multicenter, retrospective, observational study of the clinical outcomes and risk factors for relapse of ulcerative colitis at 1 year after leukocytapheresis. Journal of Gastroenterology. 2018;**53**(3):387-396. DOI: 10.1007/s00535-017-1356-8

[72] Ozeki K, Tanida S, Mizoshita T, et al. Combination therapy with intensive granulocyte and monocyte adsorptive apheresis plus adalimumab: Therapeutic outcomes in 5 cases with refractory Crohn's disease. Case Reports in Gastroenterology. 2012;**6**(3):765-771. DOI: 10.1159/000346312

[73] Naganuma M, Yokoyama Y, Motoya S, et al. Efficacy of apheresis as maintenance therapy for patients with ulcerative colitis in an open-label prospective multicenter randomised controlled trial. J Gastroenterol. 2020;**55**(4):390-400. DOI: 10.1007/s00535-019-01651-0

[74] Rodríguez-Lago I, Benítez JM, García-Sánchez V, et al. Granulocyte and monocyte apheresis in inflammatory bowel disease: The patients' point of view. Gastroenterología y Hepatología. 2018;**41**(7):423-431. DOI: 10.1016/j.gastrohep.2018.04.007

[75] Sawada K, Ohdo M, Ino T, et al. Safety and tolerability of nafamostat mesilate and heparin as anticoagulants in leukocytapheresis for ulcerative colitis: Post hoc analysis of a large-scale, prospective, observational study. Therapeutic Apheresis and Dialysis. 2016;**20**(2):197-204. DOI: 10.1111/1744-9987.12357

[76] Fukunaga K, Kamikozuru K, Yokoyama Y, et al. Optimal apheresis treatment volume for the efficacy and safety of leukocytapheresis with Cellsorba in patients with active

ulcerative colitis. Journal of Clinical Apheresis. 2011;**26**(6):326-331. DOI: 10.1002/jca.20314

[77] Vecchi M, Vernia P, Riegler G, D'Incà R, Annese V, Bagnoli S. Therapeutic landscape for ulcerative colitis: Where is the Adacolumn(®) system and where should it be? Clinical and Experimental Gastroenterology. 2013;**6**:1-7. DOI: 10.2147/CEG.S33275

[78] Kruis W, Nguyen P, Morgenstern J, et al. Novel leucocyte/thrombocyte apheresis for induction of steroid-free remission in ulcerative colitis: A controlled randomized pilot study. Journal of Crohn's & Colitis. 2019;**13**(7):949-953. DOI: 10.1093/ecco-jcc/jjz005

Chapter 6

Crohn's Disease Treated by Chinese Medicine

Xiaomei Wang, Luyi Wu, Siyi Lv, Mei Li and Huangan Wu

Abstract

Crohn's disease is an inflammatory bowel disease with variable clinical symptoms, it can affect the whole gastrointestinal tract from the oral cavity to the anus and lead to lower quality of life and greater social and economicloss. Traditional Chinese medicine (TCM) has a long history and is unique characteristic by the theory of overall concept and treatment based on syndrome differentiation, it should be an important part of world medicine. This chapter introduces the research advance of Crohn's disease in TCM, including its name, location, etiology and pathogenesis, syndrome differentiation, therapeutic criteria, treatment methods and other contents. The mechanism of TCM treatment of Crohn's disease remains to be further studied.

Keywords: Crohn's disease, Chinese medicine, acupuncture and moxibustion, diagnosis, syndrome differentiation, treatment

1. Introduction

Crohn's disease (CD) is an inflammatory disease of the gut, it and ulcerative colitis is called inflammatory bowel disease (IBD). The etiology of CD is unknown that related to genetics, environment, humoral immunity and cellular immunity to some extent. It may be due to the complex interaction between genetic susceptibility, environmental factors, and changes in intestinal microflora, resulting in mucosal immune response abnormalities and impaired epithelial barrier function, giving rise to congenital and adaptive immune response disorders [1, 2].

CD is a proliferative disease that runs through all layers of the intestinal wall and it can occur anywhere in the gastrointestinal tract, the most common being the terminal ileum and colon [2, 3]. CD has various clinical manifestations, mainly characterized by diarrhea, mucous pus and blood stool, accompanied by abdominal pain, tenesmus, fever, anemia, nutritional disorders and other systemic symptoms of varying degrees. It can also be accompanied by joint, skin, eyes, oral mucosa, liver and other extraintestinal lesions, or cause perianal lesions, intestinal obstruction, gastrointestinal bleeding, perforation and other complications [4]. This disease is mainly divided into inflammatory stage, stenosis stage and perforation stage, patients usually develop from inflammation to stenosis or perforation [3]. At present, the global incidence of CD is on the rise, and the onset age is mostly between 20 and 40 years old, with no significant gender difference [5]. CD has prolonged course, repeated attacks, and not easy to cure, which seriously affects the quality of life of patients, and aggravates the social and economic burden. Therefore, it urgently needs to be solved and further studied.

In 2012, the Inflammatory Bowel Disease Group of Gastroenterology Branch of Chinese Medical Association formulated The Consensus Opinion on the Diagnosis and Treatment of Inflammatory Bowel Disease, which standardized the clinical diagnosis and treatment of CD. In recent years, with the increasing incidence of CD, in order to meet clinical needs and better guide the clinical work, the staff of the Inflammatory Bowel Disease Group of Gastroenterology Branch of Chinese Medical Association, finally revised the 2018 edition of The Consensus Opinion on the Diagnosis and Treatment of Inflammatory Bowel Disease after extensive discussions.

As the etiology of CD is unknown, there is no radical cure at present and the side effects of drugsare obvious in some CD patients. However, the advantages of Traditional Chinese medicine (TCM) in CD treatment are gradually emerging. With the in-depths of research on CD, more and more TCM doctors and scholars have summarized the etiology and pathogenesis, TCM classification, syndrome differentiation methods and treatment principles, and summarized the characteristic treatment methods of TCM, providing the diagnosis and treatment ideas and guidance for the understanding and treatment of CD.

2. Diagnosis of CD by Western medicine

The diagnosis of CD depends on a combination of symptoms, endoscopy, radiology, and histopathological findings. Colonoscopy and mucosal biopsy are usually the main methods. A history of smoking, family history, gastrointestinal infection, malnutrition or anemia are all factors that should be taken into account when making a diagnosis [1].

2.1 Clinical manifestations

The clinical presentation of CD depends on the site of pathological changes and the severity of inflammation, which can be divided into four aspects [6]:

(1) Digestive system performance: Spasmodic pain in right lower abdomen or peri-umbilicus, accompanied by borborygmus, aggravation after meals, it can be alleviated after defecation; diarrhea intermittent attacks in early stage, and more persistent in later stage. If the lesions involve the lower colon or rectum, mucinous blood stool and tenesmus may be present. Abdominal mass occurs in the right lower abdomen and around the umbilicus, mostly caused by mesenteric lymph node enlargement, internal fistula or local abscess formation. (2) General performance: Patients with intermittent low or moderate fever, a few show remittent fever, accompanied by toxemia; Nutritional disorders due to anorexia, and chronic diarrhea, including emaciation, anemia, hypoproteinemia, vitamin deficiency, calcium deficiency, osteoporosis, etc. The balance of water, electrolyte, acid and base is disturbed in acute stage. (3) Extraintestinal manifestations: Some patients have iridocyclitis, uveitis, finger pestles, arthritis, erythema nodosum gangrenous pyoderma, oral mucosal ulcer, chronic hepatitis, small bile duct peripheral inflammation, sclerosing cholangitis and so on. Amyloidosis or thromboembolic disease can be seen occasionally. (4) Perianal manifestations: Fistulas, fissures, abscesses, and stenosis around the anus or rectum [7]. It even affects the organs outside the gut.

2.2 Endoscopic examination and diagnosis

Colonoscope is the most sensitive method in the diagnosis of CD, which can improve the accuracy of clinical diagnosis and the efficiency of treatment [8]. Under endoscopy at the early stage of the disease, 2 ~ 3 mm diameter round shallow pitting ulcers or Afta aphthous ulcer can be seen with surrounding mucosa hyperemia and redness. After the disease progresses, the ulcer increases and deepens, and merges with each other to form longitudinal ulcer. The relatively specific endoscopic manifestations include cobblestone changes, annular, multiple, segmental stenosis, and inflammatory polyp hyperplasia. Capsule endoscopy is very sensitive to the judgment of abnormal mucosa, but its specificity is low, and it is not applicable to all CD patients. For patients with stenosis, there is a certain risk. Wireless video capsule endoscope has the advantages of no radiation, no pain, no sedation, easy outpatient use and high patient satisfaction. When traditional diagnostic tools such as endoscope cannot make a clear diagnosis, it can be mainly used. During the development of CD, some patients may involve the upper digestive tract. This type of CD usually presents insidiously without obvious symptoms. Gastroscopy is often used, under which worm etched ulcer, longitudinal ulcer, slub like appearance, stenosis and fistula can be seen [9].

2.3 Pathological diagnosis

Based on the principle of multi-point and multi-segment sampling, CD mucosal biopsy is the most main diagnostic basis of CD. Its pathologic findings are typically non-caseous granulomas that are more easily detected on biopsy in about 30% of cases and are more common in smaller ulcers. In addition, common pathological features include segmental lesions, the presence of inflammatory cell infiltration in the inherent membrane, and submucosal broadening, marked fibrosis, whole-wall inflammation, fissured ulcers, and whole-layer lymphatic follicles in the intestinal wall [10, 11].

2.4 Imaging diagnosis

Imaging also plays a very important role in the diagnosis of CD. CT small intestine imaging or magnetic resonance enterography is the first choice for imaging examination, which is mainly used to evaluate inflammatory lesions in the small intestine. Magnetic resonance enterography is expensive but has the advantage of avoiding radiation and using no iodized contrast agents. The use of contrast-enhanced ultrasound can effectively improve the detection sensitivity of color Doppler ultrasound, which is outstanding in the diagnosis of the combined sensitivity and specificity of CD activity [12]. The sensitivity of small intestinal barium contrast is low and only suitable for dynamic observation in patients with intestinal cavity stenosis, and for the primary medical unit cannot conduct CT small intestinal imaging examination. Barium enema is not used much at present and has been replaced by colonoscopy.

2.5 Laboratory examination and diagnosis

The blood counts are used to monitor anemia in CD patients. The concentration of calcium protective protein in feces was associated with neutrophil infiltration in the intestinal mucosa, it has a strong sensitivity and specificity for CD diagnosis. As an inflammation marker, C-reactive protein and other inflammatory markers are used simultaneously to monitor disease activity to assess disease activity.

3. TCM diagnosis of CD

Although there is no corresponding name of CD in ancient Chinese medical books, there are abundant discussions about it, so the TCM diagnosis of CD was mainly based on symptom diagnosis. According to the main symptoms, CD is diagnosed as abdominal pain, diarrhea, bowel carbuncle, hemafecia, anal fistula, spouting bleeding from anus and other diseases [13, 14].

4. TCM etiology and pathogenesis of CD

4.1 Etiology

CD is associated with a number of pathogenic factors, either alone or in combination. Exogenous pathogenic factors, improper diet, emotional disorders, chronic physical deficiency were the main causes [14]. Exogenous pathogenic factors, such as cold, dampness and heat invade the body, resulting in blood stasis and abdominal pain and diarrhea. Unclean food, or overeating, or eating greasy and cold food can cause damp-heat or cold-dampness accumulating in stomach and spleen, blockage of abdomen Qi, producing diarrhea, bowel carbuncle; Internal injury of emotions, such as moodiness and worry leads to stagnation of qi induce pain easily; Weakness, prolonged illness or excessive fatigue, resulting in weakness of the spleen and stomach, transport and transformation weak that induce abdominal pain and diarrhea. CD mainly occurs in the intestine. In the theory of TCM, CD is also closely related to the spleen, stomach, liver and kidney, and is mainly caused by lesions in middle-jiao and lower-jiao.

4.2 Pathogenesis

The basic pathogenesis of CD is a mixture of deficiency and excess, cold and heat [15]. The deficient root include the deficiency of natural endowments, the deficiency of spleen and kidney, or the prolonged illness and overwork; Damp-heat accumulation, qi stagnation, phlegm and dampness, blood stasis are all belong to excessive superficial. The basic pathogenesis of CD varies according to the main symptoms. If abdominal pain is the main manifestation, the basic pathogenesis is exogenous pathogenic factors of coldness, wetness, heat, it result in qi stagnation, blood stasis, viscera and qi adverse, pain [16]; If the main manifestation is diarrhea, the basic pathogenesis is spleen deficiency and overabundance of dampness [16, 17]; If the main manifestation is intestinal carbuncle, the pathogenesis includes accumulation of dampness and heat, blood stasis, and the accumulation of phlegm and blood stasis [14].

5. TCM syndrome differentiation and treatment of CD

According to the Guidelines of Traditional Chinese Medicine Diagnosis and Treatment of Digestive Diseases compiled by the Committee of Spleen-stomach Diseases of The Chinese Association of TCM in 2006, the common TCM syndromes of CD include the syndrome of liver-stagnation and spleen-deficiency, the syndrome of deficiency and cold of spleen and stomach, the syndrome of yang deficiency of spleen and kidney, the syndrome of cold-dampness impairing spleen splenic function, the syndrome of qi stagnation and blood stasis syndrome, the syndrome of damp-heat accumulation [18, 19].

5.1 Syndrome of liver-stagnation and spleen-deficiency

The main symptoms are anorexia, belching, right abdominal pain or periumbilical distension pain and diarrhea while during abdominal pain and relief of pain after diarrhea. Acute abdominal pain, loose stools, belching and eat less, tongue reddish, and pulsed strings. Its attacks or exacerbations are often caused by irritation or nervous tension. The principle of treatment is soothing the liver and strengthening the spleen. The main prescriptions are Chaihu Shugan powder and Shenlinbaizhu powder [20] including bupleurum, *Codonopsis pilosula*, poria cocos, Chinese yam, white lablab album, atractylodes macrocephala koidz, fructus aurantii, lotus seed, amomum, coix seed, rhizoma cyperi, pericarpium citri reticulatae, raidix paeoniae alba, platycodon grangdiflorum, radix glycyrrhizae. Patients with anorexia can add fried hawthorn, malt; Patients with nausea and vomiting can add pinellia ternate, inula flower.

5.2 Syndrome deficiency and cold of spleen and stomach

The main symptoms are dull abdominal pain, prefer warm and pressing, prolonged diarrhea, bowel bloating and abdominal distension, vomiting of clear water, loss of appetite, sallow complexion, dizziness, cold limbs, fatigue, pale tongue, thin and white coating, and slow and sunken pulse. The principle of treatment is to warm stomach and strengthen spleen. The main prescription is Shenling Baizhu powder and Fuzi Lizhong pill [21], including fried semen coicis, fried atractylodes macrocephala koidz, poria cocos, *Codonopsis pilosula*, radix paeoniae alba, lotus seed, Chinese yam, bupleurum, giant typhonium rhizome (decocted first), corydalis yanhusuo, common bletilla pseudobulb, amomum (decocted later), honey-fried radix liquiritiae, dried ginger, panax notoginseng powder (take with water). Patient with frequency of defecation can be added nutmeg, *Terminalia chebula*; Patient with bloody stool can be added roasted ginger charcoal, patient with mucus stool can be added atractylodes.

5.3 Syndrome of deficiency of spleen and kidney yang

The main symptoms are dull abdominal pain, irregular pain attacks and stop, prefer warm and pressing, thin pus around the anus, dull anal pain, loose stool, or diarrhea at dawn, loss of appetite, fatigue, cold limbs, soreness of waist and polyuria, pale tongue, or fat tongue with teeth marks, white coating, sunken or or thin and weak pulse. The principle of treatment is warming kidney and strengthening spleen. The main prescription is Changyangan soup [22], including astragalus membranaceus, poria cocos, *Codonopsis pilosula*, rhizoma bletillae, pseudo-ginseng, cooked monkshood, fructus psoraleae, *Myristica fragrans*, epimedium, fructus chebulae, radix glycyrrhizae.

5.4 Syndrome of cold dampness impairing spleen

The main symptoms are acute abdominal pain, loose stool or water stool, or dysentery with blood and pus, heavy head and body, pale tongue, white and greasy coating, soft and slow pulse. The principle of treatment is clearing damp and strengthening spleen. The main prescription is Weiling soup, including atractylodes rhizome, dried tangerine peel, magnolia officinalis, polyporus umbellatus, rhizoma alismatis, cortex cinnamomi, atractylodes macrocephala koidz, radix glycyrrhizae.

5.5 Syndrome of qi stagnation and blood stasis

The main symptoms are immovable abdominal lumps, abdominal distension or pricking, loose or bloody stools, purplish or petechial tongue, string and thin and hesitant pulse. The principle of treatment is regulating qi and dispersing blood stasis. The main prescription is infradiaphragmatic stasis-expelling decoction, including peach kernel, safflower, radix rehmanniae, radix angelicae sinensis, red peony, fructus aurantii, *Platycodon grandiflorum*, radix glycyrrhizae, radix bupleuri, radix scrophulariae.

5.6 Syndrome of damt-heat accumulation

The main symptoms are abdominal pain refusing to press, brown and smelly stool, or diarrhea with blood and pus, distending pain and scorching hot anus, thirsty and drinking cold, few and yellow urine, red tongue, yellow greasy coating, string and slippery or slippery and rapid pulse. The treatment principle is clearing heat and expelling damp. The main prescription is Baitouweng soup, including pulsatilla, coptis chinensis, phellodendron, ash bark.

Chinese herbal medicine.

Name	Pharmacological effects
Bupleurum	Diaphoresis; prevent malaria
Codonopsis pilosula	enrich blood; immunity enhancement
Poria cocos	Calm; promote healthy digestion
Chinese yam	Improve immune and digestive function
White lablab bean	Antibacterial and antiviral
Atractylodes macrocephala koidz	Adjust gastrointestinal motility; inhibit ulcer
Fructus aurantii	Increases gastrointestinal motility and contractility rhythms
Lotus seed	Immune regulation; improve digestive function
Amomum	bacteriostatic action; peristalsis enhancement
Coix seed	Eliminate edema; immune regulation
Rhizoma cyperi	Relaxes intestinal smooth muscle; anti-inflammatory
Pericarpium citri reticulatae	Promote secretion of digestive juices; relieve asthma
Raidix paeoniae alba	Antibacterial activity; analgesic
Platycodon grangdiflorum	Dilate blood vessels; antitussive expectorant
Radix glycyrrhizae	Regulate immunity; inhibit ulcer; protect liver
Fried hawthorn	Help digestion; stop diarrhea
Malt	Help digestion; antifungal
Pinellia ternate	Antitussive expectorant; inhibit ulcer
Inula flower	Relieve asthma; antitussive expectorant
Giant typhonium rhizome	Anti-inflammatory; sedation; expectorant
Corydalis yanhusuo	Spasmolysis, analgesia; suppression of gastric ulcer
Common bletilla pseudobulb	Hemostasis; protect gastric mucosa
Dried ginger	Inhibit ulcer; dilate blood vessels
Panax notoginseng powder	Promote blood clotting; dilate blood vessels
Nutmeg	Antibacteria; anti-inflammatory
Terminalia chebula	Antibacteria; antitumor; antidiarrhea
Roasted ginger charcoal	Hemostasis; acesodyne
Atractylodes	Adjust gastrointestinal motility; diuresis
Astragalus membranaceus	Strengthen immune system; inhibit ulcer; improve substance metabolism
Cooked monkshood	Cardiac; antishock; dilate blood vessels
Fructus psoraleae	Antibacteria; improve immune system
Epimedium	Improve immune system; delay the progression of renal failure

Name	Pharmacological effects
Magnolia officinalis	Promote the secretion of digestive fluids; anti ulcer
Polyporus umbellatus	Diuresis; enhance immunity
Rhizoma alismatis	Diuresis; anti-inflammatory
Cortex cinnamomi	Cardiotonic; anti ulcer; anti-inflammatory
Peach kernel	Reduce vascular resistance and improve hemodynamics; relax bowels
Safflower	Dilate blood vessels; excited uterus; anticoagulation
Radix rehmanniae	Hemostasis; antibiosis; immuno-enhancement
Radix angelicae	Anti-microbico; Antipyretic analgesic
Sinensis	Promote hematopoietic function; immunity enhancement
Red peony	Antithrombus; reduce blood lipid; liver protection
Radix scrophulariae	Antibiosis; dilate coronary arteries
Pulsatilla	Anti-microbico; anti-inflammatory; immunity enhancement
Coptis chinensis	Resistance of pathogens; Antipyretic; antineoplastic
Phellodendron	anti-microbico; excite gastrointestinal smooth muscle
Ash bark	Anti-inflammatory; analgesic; diuresis

6. Chinese patent medicines

A large number of studies and clinical evidence show that TCM has obvious curative effect and function in the treatment of CD. The following is a brief summary of commonly used Chinese patent medicines.

6.1 Bolus for strengthening intestines and relieving diarrhea

It has the effect of harmonizing liver and spleen, astringent intestine to relieve pain [23] and commonly used in patients with disharmony of liver and spleen, diarrhea and abdominal pain, and nonspecific ulcerative colitis.

6.2 Salvia ligustrazin injection

It has the effect of activating blood circulation and removing blood stasis, improving microcirculation. The cure rate can be improved by improving the high coagulation state of CD patients [24].

6.3 Warming kidney and invigorating spleen granules

It has the effect of strenthening spleen and tonifying kidney. It can improve the humoral immunity of patients also used todiseases caused by the deficiency of spleen and kidney.

6.4 Tripterygium wilfordii polyglycoside tablet

It has the effect of dispelling wind and detoxifying, dehumidifying and detumescence, relaxing tendons and dredging collaterals. Studies have shown that it can effectively improve the clinical symptoms of CD patient [25], but its toxicity of liver and kidney should be valued.

6.5 Sishen pill

It has the effect of warming kidney and dispelling cold, astringent intestine and relieving diarrhea and commonly used for diarrhea caused by deficiency of kidney yang, the symptoms are borborygmus, intestinal distension, diarrhea at dawn, anorexia and indigestion, continuous diarrhea, yellowish complexion and cold limbs.

6.6 Dark plum pill

It has the effect of smoothing liver and regulating intestine, clearing the upper Jiao and warming lower Jiao and used for patient with chronic dysentery, the symptoms are abdominal pain, dysentery, vertex headache, attack intermittently, irritation and vomiting, extremities cold.

6.7 Peaceful gastroenterology tablets

It has the effect of invigorating spleen and kidney, warming stomach and relieving pain, astringent intestine and relieving diarrhea, and used for patient with diarrhea of deficiency of spleen and kidney Yang, the symptoms are irregular stool, diarrhea at dawn with mucus, abdominal distention and pain, epigastric discomfort, and distention of lower abdominal.

6.8 Buzhong Yiqi pill

It has the effect of invigorating and benefiting spleen qi and lifting collapsed qi, be used for diarrhea caused by weakness of spleen and stomach and collapse of middle qi.

6.9 Guben Yichang tablets

It has the effect of invigorating spleen and warming kidney, astringing intestine to relieve diarrhea, and be used for chronic diarrhea caused by spleen deficiency or Yang deficiency of spleen-kidney, the symptoms are chronic abdominal pain and diarrhea, loose stools, anorexia and abdominal distension, weak waist, fatigue and cold limbs.

6.10 Aucklandia and coptis tablets

It has the effect of clearing away heat and eliminating dampness, promoting qi circulation to relieve pain, and be used for dysentery caused by dampness-heat of large intestine, the symptoms are stool with pus and blood, tenesmus, fever and abdominal pain.

6.11 Fuzi Lizhong pill

It has the effect of warming spleen dispersing cold, relieving diarrhea and pain, and can be used for cold syndrome of spleen and stomach, the symptoms are anorexia and abdominal distension, abdominal pain and nausea, weak pulse, cold limbs, or headache attacked by cold, and any chronic disease caused by cold.

6.12 Zhuche pill

It has the effect of nourishing Yin and blood, tonifying qi and strong intestine, removing blood stasis and generating muscles. The symptoms are dull abdominal pain, persistent diarrhea, stool with pus and blood, low fever in afternoon, dizziness, insomnia, night sweats, irritability, weight loss and fatigue, red tongue, thin and less coating, thin and rapid pulse.

7. Acupuncture and moxibusiton treatment of CD

Acupuncture therapy is widely applicable to mild and moderate CD patient with no age or gender restrictions, but not for patients with severe CD, in pregnancy and lactation, with mental disorders, with severe tumors, or patients with serious diseases of the heart, liver, kidney, brain and hematopoietic system [26], they need adopt appropriate western medicine to save lives and avoid critical situations.

The basic acupoint prescriptions for CD treatment include Tianshu (ST25), Zusanli (ST36), Shangjuxu (ST37), Guanyuan (RN4), Qihai (RN6), Zhongwan (RN12) [27]. Patients with syndrome of liver depression and spleen deficiency can add Taichong (LR3) and Pishu (BL20); Patients with syndrome of deficiency and cold of spleen and stomach can add Shangwan (RN13) and Xiawan (RN10); Patients with syndrome of yang deficiency of spleen and kidney were added with Mingmen (DU4), Pishu (BL20) and Shenshu (BL23); Patients with syndrome of cold dampness disturbing spleencan add Yanglingquan (GB34) and Fenglong (ST40); Patients with syndrome of qi stagnation and blood stasis can add Taichong (LR3) and Qihai (SP10); Patients with syndrome of dampness-heat accumulation can add Quchi (LI11) and Hegu (LI4). During the acupuncture treatment, the abdomen of CD patients is usually the main part, including the legs and back. The treatment is normally performed for about 20-30 minutes each time, once every other day. If the patient is in serious condition, the curative effect can be enhanced once a day.

Acupuncture therapy is mainly targeted at excess, heat syndrome and relatively simple symptom. For patients with syndrome of intermingled deficiency and excess, acupuncture therapy often combines with moxibustion therapy. The research of Wu Huangan research group showed [28, 29] that moxibustion can effectively improve the clinical symptoms and the quality of life of CD patient. The methods were mainly acupuncture at Tianshu (ST25), Zhongwan (RN12), Qihai (RN6). Mix the powder of aconite, cinnamon, salvia miltiorrhiza, safflower, costusroot, coptis chinensis and borneol; add yellow rice wine and mix it to form a thick paste; Make a medical cake in a mold and place it at the above acupoints, and place moxa cone on medical cake, moxibustion twice for each acupoint; Combined with acupuncture at Zusanli (ST36), Shangjuxu (ST37), Sanyinjiao (SP6) and Gongsun (SP4), the goal of synergetic treatment and enhanced curative effect was finally achieved.

8. Other therapies

In addition to TCM, Chinese patent medicine, acupuncture and moxibustion treatment methods, there are other unique therapies, and the effect is also very effective. Through clinical controlled experiments, Songnian proved [30] that auricular application can effectively alleviate the abdominal pain of CD patients. Enema administration combined with internal medicine can greatly improve the curative effect of CD [31]. Hu Zhengchao and et al. [32] have found that Chinese medicine fumigation, external washing and sitz bath could effectively alleviate the symptoms of anal fistula patients with CD, not only improving local blood circulation, but promoting the healing of anal fistula canal. In addition, fecal flora transplantation is also a new treatment method for CD combined with Chinese medicine, it works by transplanting fecal material from a healthy donor into the patient's gut to restore the intestinal flora diversity and thus achieve a good therapeutic effect [33].

9. Criteria of efficacy evaluation

9.1 Crohn's disease activity index (CDAI)

CDAI can be used to evaluate the disease activity and the efficacy of CD, including five aspects of the patient's general condition, such as abdominal pain, diarrhea, abdominal mass and complications [34]. The higher the total score, the more serious the disease. A score of ≤4 indicates remission, a score of 5-8 indicates moderate activity, and a score of ≥9 indicates severe activity. It can be scored in three stages before, during and after treatment to dynamically observe the changes of the disease.

9.2 Overall efficacy of TCM syndromes

The total score of TCM syndromes was used to evaluate the clinical symptoms of abdominal pain, diarrhea, pus and blood stool, tenesmus, belching, nausea and vomiting and fever. The total scores before and after treatment was compared, if the total score decreased by ≥90% compared with that before treatment, it is judged as clinical remission. If the total score decreased by ≥70% and < 90%, it is judged as significant effect; if the total score decreased ≥30%and < 70%, it is judged to be valid; if the total score decreased <30%, it is judged to be invalid.

9.3 Endoscopic score

Simplified endoscopy score for CD (SESCD) can be used for diagnosis and efficacy evaluation of CD. The score items mainly include ulcer size, ulcer area, affected intestinal area, intestinal lumen stenosis and the condition of mucosal healing. The lower the score, the better the mucosal healing degree. A score ≤ 3 is remission, a score 4-10 is mild activity, a score 11-19 is moderate activity, and a score more than 20 is severe activity [35].

9.4 Quality of life assessment

Inflammatory bowel disease quality of life questionnaire (IBDQ) was used for CD evaluation, including intestinal symptoms, systemic symptoms, emotional ability and social ability. Scores were recorded for both the pre-treatment and post-treatment stages, with higher scores indicating better quality of life.

9.5 Assessment of anxiety and depression

Self-rating anxiety scale (SAS) and self-rating depression scale (SDS) were used to evaluate the severity of the anxiety and the depressive symptoms of CD patients. Scores were performed according to the symptoms, and the patients were divided into mild, moderate and severe by 50 score. Scores were recorded before and after treatment. Scores below 50 after treatment indicated efficacy.

9.6 Long-term efficacy

The development of CD is a long-term and progressive process. The clinical efficacy evaluation should combine the short-term with long-term efficacy. In addition to the general clinical symptoms, it is also important to observe the status with the ulcer of intestinal mucosa and actively prevent perianal lesions it should also focus on the observation of intestinal mucosal ulcer and the active prevention of perianal lesions of CD patients.

10. Prevention and care

10.1 Diet control

Improper diet is one of the major causes of CD. In TCM, dampness, heat and cold pathogens easily invade the body through improper diet, damage spleen and stomach, and accumulate in intestines. Therefore, CD patients should pay attention to their daily diet, light and easy digestible food is better, avoid eat irritating food, try not to eat or eat less fat and greasy food, or raw and cold food.

10.2 Psychological adjustment

CD is a chronic disease in the developing course of disease, patients are prone to anxiety or depression that aggravating the symptoms of body and mind. Therefore, in the process of diagnosis and treatment, attention should be paid to the psychological and emotional intervention of the patients to avoid negative emotional stimuli, relieve their anxiety or depression situation, guide the correct understanding of disease with good positive attitude [36, 37].

10.3 Adjust lifestyle

CD is persistent and prone to relapse, so it is important to adjust lifestyle, control risk factors and change improper habits. Smoking is an important factor for CD patient, which often aggravates the disease and more likely to cause complications. For CD patients, the first step is to quit smoking, adjust lifestyle, and eliminate risk factors. In addition, patients should have regular daily life, reasonable work and rest, moderate diet, maintain the spleen and stomach, do proper exercise, avoid fatigue, adjust emotions, comply with four seasons, and maintain healthy energy [38].

10.4 Regular review and follow-up

The development of CD is a long-term process, attention should always be paid to physical changes through outpatient, inpatient follow-up, telephone follow-up, and regular review, to understand the recurrence of disease, cancer prevention.

11. Conclusion

The cause of CD is still unclear, it is mainly related to improper diet, disorder emotion, attack of external evil, internal deficiency in TCM theory. The main pathogenesis is deficiency of spleen and kidney combined with damp-heat accumulation, qi stagnation, phlegm and dampness and blood stasis. The holistic concept and syndrome differentiation are the general principles of TCM treatment, the diagnostic criteria of CD are generally accorded to the consensus Opinions on the Diagnosis and Treatment of Inflammatory Bowel Disease as the reference, and comprehensive judgments are mainly made based on the clinical symptoms, endoscopy results, imaging examinations and pathological tissues of the patients. For example, the concentration of fecal calprotectin was positively correlated with CDAI score, SEC-CD score, CD clinical activity and mucosal healing, it could objectively reflect the inflammatory activity of CD [39]. Imaging diagnostic techniques, magnetic resonance imaging (MRI) and computerized tomography (CT), can be used to assess the activity of CD by showing changes in the thickness of the intestinal wall, abnormal intensification of the intestinal wall, intestinal segment stenosis, abnormal increase in mesenteric vessels, enlarged lymph nodes, fistulas, ulcers, and abscesses [40]. According to the symptoms and characteristics of different syndroms of CD, corresponding treatment methods were adopted, among which Chinese herbal medicine and acupuncture and moxibustion treatment were the most common and had significant curative effects.

With the development of TCM treatment of CD in recent years, certain progress and achievements have been made in clinical and experimental research, such as the gray matter structure of CD patients had significant changes, which was correlated with anxiety and depression status and course of disease [41]. In resting-state, the brain abnormal activities in insula and MCC of CD patients are different between remissive CD patients with and without abdominal pain, and are closely related to the severity of abdominal pain [42], aberrant functional connectivity of the amygdala may be involved in processing of visceral pain and sensation, and emotion in CD [43]. Herb-partition moxibustion combined with acupuncture can improve the clinical common symptoms of abdominal pain, diarrhea, fatigue and anorexia for mild and moderate CD [26]. Both treatments of electro-acupuncture and moxibustion improved cortex-subcortical coupling in remissive CD patients, but electro-acupuncture regulated homeostatic afferent processing network, while moxibustion mainly regulated the default mode network [44]. In CD rats, moxibustion can up-regulate the A20 expression level and down-regulate the expression of TNFR1, TRADD, and RIP1, and increase cell apoptosis in the intestinal epithelial barrier [45]. It is important to relieve the damage of intestinal mucosal barrier and maintain its functional integrity for patients [46]. Many experimental studies have shown that moxibustion can significantly down-regulate the expression of NF - κB P65, TNF-α and IL-1 in the colon tissue of CD model rats [47] and down-regulate the proteins expression of MCP-1 and IL-8 to reduce the expression of downstream inflammatory factors, relieve intestinal inflammation, and improve the morphological structure of colon tissue [48].

However, the pathogenesis of CD is still unclear, there is a lack of prospective studies even large sample and multicenter clinical trials, which still need to be further studied and explored.

Acknowledgements

Authors thank the Inflammatory Bowel Disease Group of Gastroenterology Branch of Chinese Medical Association for the Consensus opinions of TCM diagnosis and treatment experts on Crohn's disease.

Authors thank for the support of National Basic Research Programme of China (973 programme, grant number 2015CB554501).

Conflict of interest

There is no conflict of interest among authors.

Author details

Xiaomei Wang*, Luyi Wu, Siyi Lv, Mei Li and Huangan Wu
Shanghai University of Traditional Chinese Medicine, Shanghai, China

*Address all correspondence to: wxm123@vip.sina.com

References

[1] Torres J, Mehandru S, Colombel JF, Peyrin-Biroulet L. Crohn's disease. Lancet. 2017 Apr 29;389(10080):1741-1755. doi:10.1016/S0140-6736(16)31711-1. Epub 2016 Dec 1. PMID: 27914655.

[2] Veauthier B, Hornecker JR. Crohn's Disease: Diagnosis and Management. Am Fam Physician. 2018 Dec 1;98(11):661-669. PMID: 30485038.

[3] Feuerstein JD, Cheifetz AS. Crohn Disease: Epidemiology, Diagnosis, and Management. Mayo Clin Proc. 2017 Jul;92(7):1088-1103. doi: 10.1016/j.mayocp.2017.04.010. PMID: 28601423.

[4] Guo YH, Niu WW, Zhang XL. Intelpretation of the consensus on diagnosis and management of inflammatory bowel diseases (Beijing, 2018) from the perspective of diagnosis of Crohn's disease. Clinical Focus, 2018,33(12):1077-1079.

[5] Gajendran M, Loganathan P, Catinella AP, et al. A comprehensive review and update on Crohn's disease. Dis Mon. 2018 Feb;64(2):20-57. doi: 10.1016/j.disamonth.2017.07.001. PMID: 28826742.

[6] Consensus on diagnosis and Treatment of Inflammatory Bowel Disease (Beijing, 2018). Chinese Journal of Inflammatory Bowel Disease, 2018(03): 173-190.

[7] Zalieckas JM. Treatment of perianal Crohn's disease. Semin Pediatr Surg. 2017 Dec;26(6):391-397. doi: 10.1053/j.sempedsurg.2017.10.009. PMID: 29126509.

[8] Yao P, Zheng YN, Xin YJ, et al. Application of digestive endoscopy in the diagnosis and treatment of inflammatory bowel disease. Journal of Colorectal & Anal Surgery, 2020,26(S1):26-27.

[9] Chen YY, Zhao L (reviewing), Wang FY, et al. Clinical characteristics, diagnosis and treatment status and analysis of Crohn's disease with upper gastrointestinal tract phenotype. Military Medical Journal of Southeast China, 2020,22(4):385-389.

[10] Zhang M, Fu YJ, Jiang ZN. Pathological differential diagnosis of Crohn's disease. Modern Practical Medicine, 2020,32(7):746-749+738.

[11] Ouyang Q, Liang HL. Crohn's disease. Continuing medical education, 2006,20(3):35-39.

[12] Tang XY, Xuan JQ, Li X, et al. Diagnostic value of contrast-enhanced ultrasonography for active Crohn' s disease: a systematic review and Meta-analysis. Journal of Clinical Ultrasound in Medicine, 2020,22(6):429-434.

[13] Zhu GJ. New Research Progress on the Treatment of Crohn's Disease by Traditional Chinese Medicine. World Latest Medicine Information, 2019(46):112-113.

[14] Li MX, Zhao WX. Etiology and Pathogenesis of Crohn's Disease in Traditional Chinese Medicine. Journal of Shandong University of TCM,2020,44(4):396-399.

[15] Chen JF. Chinese medicine syndrome treatment of Crohn's disease. Guiding Journal of Traditional Chinese Medicine and Pharmacy, 2017,23(5):9-11.

[16] Fang GD, Zhu JH. Discussion on the diagnosis and treatment of Crohn's disease from the development of diarrhea theory in Huangdi Neijing. China Journal of Traditional Chinese Medicine and Pharmacy, 2020,35(3):1412-1414.

[17] Chen Y. Advances in the treatment of Crohn's disease based on syndrome

differentiation and acupuncture. Journal of Emergency in Traditional Chinese Medicine, 2019,28(7):1313-1316.

[18] Wang YY, Zhang C, Liu HH, et al. Research progress of Traditional Chinese medicine in treating Crohn's disease. Hunan Journal of Traditional Chinese Medicine, 2018,34(11):168-170.

[19] Zhu MJ, Wang L, Yang HP. Advances in clinical research on Traditional Chinese medicine treatment of Crohn's disease. Traditional Chinese Medicinal Research, 2020,33(1):74-77.

[20] Song LX, Luo MH. Effects of chaihu shugan powder and shenling baizhu powder on nutritional status and immune function of Crohn's disease with stagnation of liver-QI with deficiency of the spleen. Journal of Qiqihar Medical University, 2019,40(12):1493-1495.

[21] Zhang M, Zhang XD, Xia YX, et al. Clinical Study on Shenling Baizhu Powder Combined with Fuzi Lizhong Pills and Western Medicine in the Treatment of Crohn's Disease. Journal of new Chinese Medicine, 2019,51(12):73-76.

[22] Wang YF, Zhu SD. Observation of Clinical Efficacy of Yanghe Decoction on Treating Crohn's Disease of Spleen-kidney Yang Deficiency Syndrome. Journal of Shandong University of TCM, 2017,41(2):138-140.

[23] Guo Y, Wei XJ, Wang YX. Clinical Effects of Guchang Zhixie Pills Combined with Mesalazine on Mildly active Crohn's disease. Chinese Traditional Patent Medicine, 2019,41(8):1844-1847.

[24] Han LK, Di YJ, Chang H. Study on Danshen Chuanxiongqin injection in treatment for inflammatory bowel disease. Modern Journal of Integrated Modern Journal of Integrated Traditional Chinese and Western Medicine, 2010,19(30):3230-3231.

[25] Zheng Y, Tao QS, Ji ZL, et al. Study on the therapeutic effect of Tripterygium wilfordii polyglycosides on rat model of Crohn's disease. Chinese Journal of General Surgery, 2013,22(12):1650-1654.

[26] Bao CH, Wu LY, Wu HG, et al. Active Crohn's disease treated with acupuncture and moxibustion: a randomized controlled trial. Zhongguo Zhen Jiu. 2016 Jul 12;36(7):683-688. PMID: 29231405.

[27] Ji QQ, Hou XF, Zhong Y, et al. Analysis on the rule of main acupoints application in acupuncture and moxibustion treatment for inflammatory bowel diseases based on data mining method. Journal of Shanxi University of Chinese Medicine, 2020,21(3):161-165.

[28] Bao Ch, Shi Y, Ma XP, et al. Pathogenesis of Crohn Disease, Advances in its Acupuncture-moxibustion Treatment and Thinking. Shanghai Journal of Acupuncture and Moxibustion, 2010,29(11):681-686.

[29] Shi Y, Bao CH, Wu HG. WU Huan-gan's experience in treating Crohn's disease based on theory of warming spleen and stomach and invigorating the kidney for dredging channels. China Journal of Traditional Chinese Medicine and Pharmacy, 2016,31(3):878-880.

[30] Song N. Observation on the Effect of Traditional Chinese medicine acupoint sticking combined with ear acupoint seed burying in relieving abdominal pain of Crohn's disease patients. Chinese General Practice Nursing, 2017,15(24):2984-2985.

[31] Xie ZX. Herbal Oral Administration and Enema Therapy of 22 Cases with Crohn's Disease. Systems Medicine, 2018,3(18):146-148.

[32] Hu ZC, Gu GS, Li GW, et al. Therapeutic Effects of Traditional Chinese Medicine Lotion in Treatment of Anal Fistula in Crohn's Disease. Clinical Journal of Traditional Chinese Medicine, 2017,29(4):568-571.

[33] Liu SL, Huang LZ, Jinag XF, et al. Application and progress of fecal flora transplantation in the treatment of inflammatory reactive bowel disease. Jilin Medical Journal, 2019,40(2):363-365.

[34] You LL,Yao YY, Lu M, et al. Current situation and influencing factors of coping style in patients with inflammatory bowel disease. Guangxi Medical Journal, 2020,42(9):1165-1170.

[35] Yuan BS, Jin XX, Lu YK, et al. Correlation between Simplified Endoscopic Score for Crohn's Disease(SES— CD) and Clinical and Laboratory Markers in Patients with Crohn's Diseas. Chinese Journal of Gastroenterology, 2017,22(3):157-162.

[36] Zhang X. Effect of psychological nursing on anxiety and depression in the patients with Crohn's disease. China Modern Doctor, 2018,56(33):137-139.

[37] Zeng X, Ye XH, Sun L, et al. Health-related quality of life of patients with Crohn's disease: A meta synthesis of qualitative studies. Journal of Medical Postgraduates, 2019,32(8):858-860.

[38] Zhang XM, Cai DB, Liu BF. Application of the idea of curing disease prevention and treatment of Crohn's disease. Hebei Chinese Medicine, 2019,41(10):1563-1565.

[39] Chen Q. The relationship between fecal calprotectin and Crohn's disease and its TCM syndromes. Zhejiang University of Traditional Chinese Medicine, 2019.

[40] Zhu J, Xu JR, Zhu ZY, et al. 3.0T MRI for assessment of disease activity in Crohn's disease. Modern Digestion & Intervention, 2010,15(04):199-204+217.

[41] Bao CH, Liu P, Liu HR, et al. Alterations in brain grey matter structures in patients with crohn's disease and their correlation with psychological distress. J Crohns Colitis. 2015 Jul;9(7):532-540. PMID: 25895879.

[42] Bao CH, Liu P, Liu HR, et al. Differences in regional homogeneity between patients with Crohn's disease with and without abdominal pain revealed by resting-state functional magnetic resonance imaging. Pain. 2016 May;157(5):1037-1044. PMID: 26761381

[43] Fan YY, Bao CH, Wei Y, et al. Altered functional connectivity of the amygdala in Crohn's disease. Brain Imaging Behav, 2020,14(6), 2097-2106. PMID: 31628591

[44] Bao C, Wang D, Liu P, et al. Effect of Electro-Acupuncture and Moxibustion on Brain Connectivity in Patients with Crohn's Disease: A Resting-State fMRI Study. Front Hum Neurosci, 2017 Nov 17;11:559. PMID: 29204113.

[45] Zhou J, Wu LY, Chen L, et al. Herbs-partitioned moxibustion alleviates aberrant intestinal epithelial cell apoptosis by upregulating A20 expression in a mouse model of Crohn's disease. World J Gastroenterol, 2019 May 7;25(17):2071-2085. PMID: 31114134.

[46] Wang K, Liu SM, Gu ME, et al. The Protection of Acupuncture & Moxibustion on Intestinal Mucosa Barrier of Crohn's Disease. Lishizhen Medicine and Materia Medica Research, 2017,28(11):2718-2721.

[47] Wei K, Zhang D, Dou CZ, et al. Study on the Regulating Effect of Moxibustion on NF－κB p65, TNF－α, and IL－1β in Colons of CD Rats. World Chinese Medicine, 2013,8(08):862-866+870.

[48] Shi Z, Zhang H, Wang XM, et al. Influence of Moxibustion on the Expressions of MCP-1 and IL-8 Proteins in the Colonic Mucosa of Crohn's Disease Rats.Shanghai Journal of Acupuncture and Moxibustion,2009,28(09):497-501.